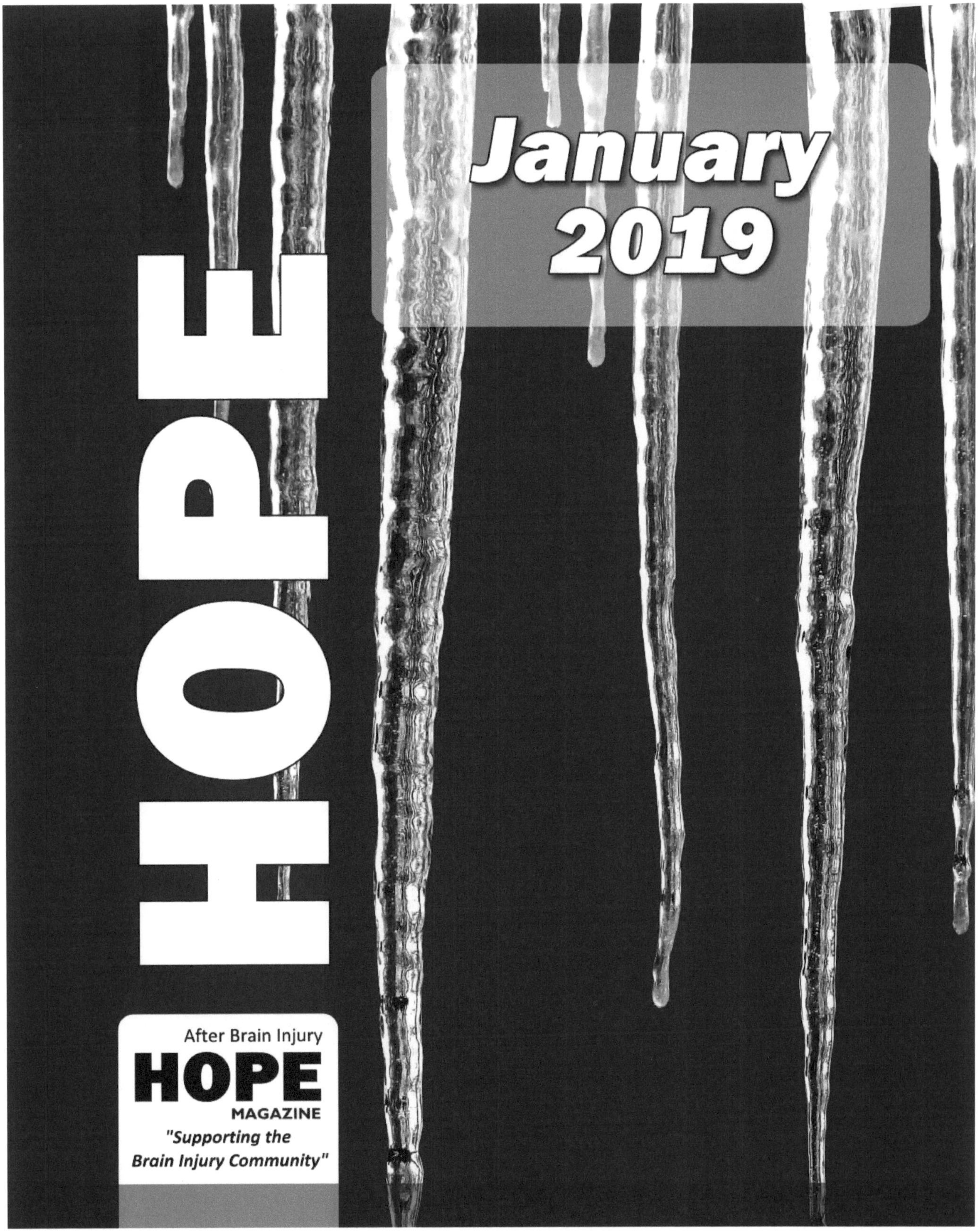

HOPE

January 2019

After Brain Injury

HOPE MAGAZINE

"Supporting the Brain Injury Community"

Welcome

HOPE MAGAZINE

Serving the Brain Injury Community

January 2019

Publisher
David A. Grant

Editor
Sarah Grant

Our Contributors

Nicole Bingaman
Patrick Brigham
Darron Eastwell
Donna Figurski
Sarah Kilch Gaffney
Rosalie Johnson
Dawne McKay
Norma Myers
Rosemary Rawlins
Jeff Sebell
Mandi Seipel
Ted Stachulski
Barbara Stahura
Carole Starr
Barbara J. Webster
Amy Zellmer

Welcome to the January 2019 issue of HOPE Magazine

This month, we bring to you what is perhaps our most amazing issue of HOPE Magazine to date. I have the high honor of introducing you to our 2019 Hope Heroes. Our heroes include writers, bloggers, family members of those affected by brain injury – and of course survivors themselves.

Each was chosen because of his or her advocacy excellence and commitment to serving others. They give of their time and resources, with no expectations other than to help others. Our January issue includes a story contributed by each of our Heroes.

It is safe to say that together as a group, these fifteen selfless souls have touched the lives of millions of people around the world. It's an amazing way to kick off another year of real hope and meaningful inspiration.

Please join me in congratulating our 2019 Hope Heroes!

Peace,

David A. Grant
Publisher

Contents

> "A hero is someone who has given his or her life to something bigger than oneself."
>
> -Joseph Campbell

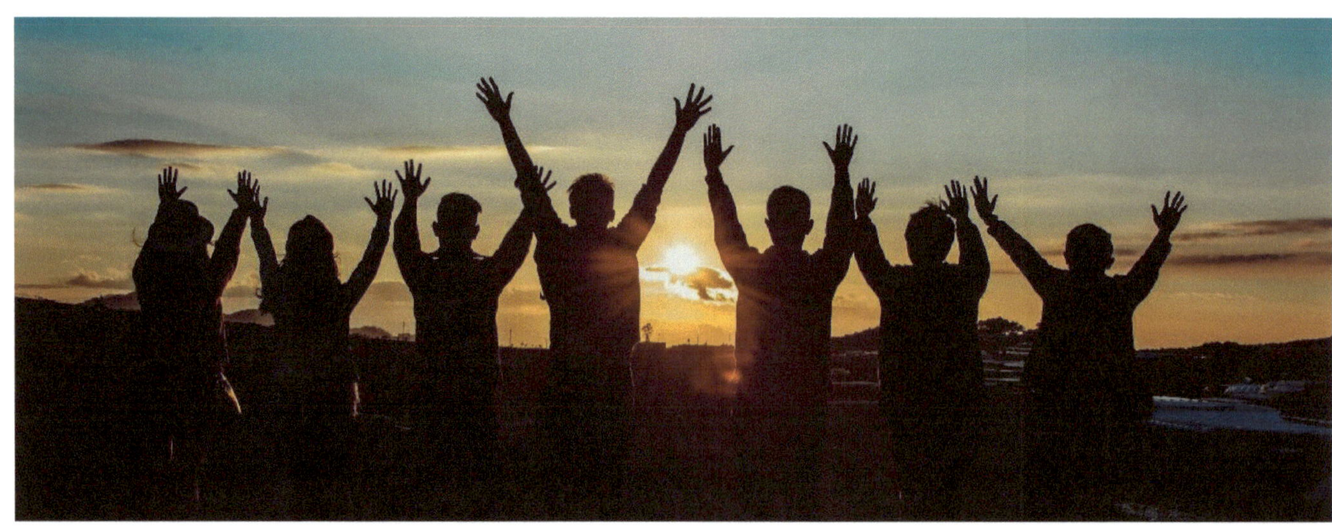

Meet the Heroes

By David A. Grant

Spanning two continents, our Hope Heroes have each, in his or her own way, said "this is not how my story will end." They have shown courage in the face of seemingly insurmountable odds and have taken what is unquestionably the toughest experience in their collective lives and turned it full-circle using their own hardship to help lift humanity higher.

Rosemary Rawlins' husband Hugh suffered a severe traumatic brain injury after a car hit him on his bike. Rosemary has served the brain injury community for many years as a tireless advocate, writer, blogger, and public speaker.

Nicole Bingaman's son Taylor suffered a traumatic brain injury after falling down a flight of stairs in 2012. Doctors said the 21-year-old would probably not live. Taylor did indeed survive. Fast forward through time, and Nicole is now a passionate family advocate, keynote presenter, and prolific writer. She knows from personal experience that love wins!

Sarah Kilch Gaffney is a writer, brain injury outreach coordinator, and works for the Maine Chapter of the *Brain Injury Association of America*. Her husband was diagnosed with a terminal brain tumor. As Sarah wrote a year-and-a-half after her husband Steve's passing, "I am still enormously hazy about what lies ahead, but I am moving forward nonetheless." And move forward she did, into a life of service to others.

Brain injury survivor **Rosalie Johnson** didn't let her own injury slow her down. Rosalie can be found running the seacoast Brain Injury Support Group in New Hampshire and volunteering at Krempels Center in Portsmouth, New Hampshire. Rosalie is also a nine-year Board Member for the *Brain Injury Association of New Hampshire*.

When a car skidded into **Barbara J. Webster**'s car on a slippery road in 1991, she didn't realize that it would lead to a new road. Barbara has served the *Brain Injury Association of Massachusetts* for many years, working within the support group community, as well as facilitating numerous workshops. She is a prolific writer and is well-loved by all who know her.

In 1999, **Carole Starr**'s life was forever changed by a motor vehicle accident. Rather than seeing it as the end of her life, Carole used her experience as a brain injury survivor to help others. Carole is the co-founder of *Brain Injury Voices,* an advocacy group, as well as a keynote presenter and published author.

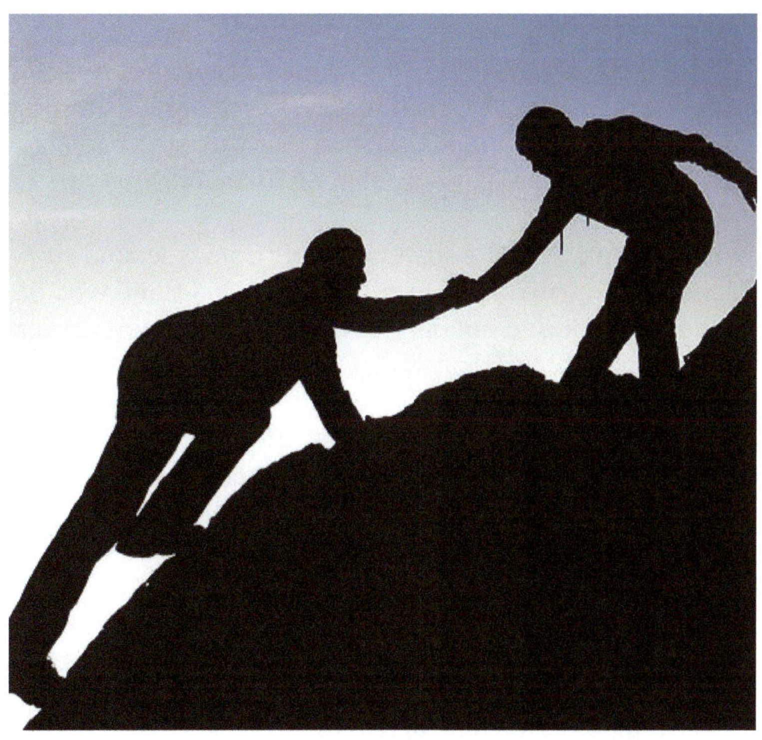

In January 2005, **Donna Figurski**'s husband, David, sustained a traumatic brain injury. Donna has steadfastly chosen to not be defeated by this tragedy. Donna has emerged as a powerful voice within the brain injury community through her radio show and has recently published a memoir about her experience.

It was a cold February day when **Amy Zellmer** slipped on a patch of sheer ice in her building's driveway, leaving Amy with a TBI. From her *Huffington Post* articles, to her vibrant social tribe, countless others have found strength in Amy's transparency, courage, and persistence.

In May of 2015, successful banking executive **Darron Eastwell** said goodbye to his wife Bianca, with plans for an exciting day of mountain biking at Tewantin National Park in Australia, never thinking that by day's end, he would sustain a brain injury. Darron has emerged as a powerful example of how life can indeed be rebuilt after brain injury. Darron is now a published author and has made countless public appearances, all in an effort to teach others about brain injury. Darron is an inspirational advocate and educator.

Dawne McKay was hit from behind by a distracted driver, causing her to be tossed around in her vehicle. She does not remember the second impact from a tractor trailer. To say that her life changed that day is an understatement. Not one to slow down, Dawne founded a social community: *Motor Vehicle Accident – Support and Recovery Group*, where she touches the lives of others around the world.

Certified Journal Facilitator, author and caregiver, **Barbara Stahura** has lived a life of service since her husband Ken's brain injury. Barbara is the co-author of the acclaimed *After Brain Injury: Telling Your Story*, the first journaling book for people with brain injury, a conference presenter, and a tireless advocate for those affected by brain injury.

Mainer **Jeff Sebell** is perhaps the most tenured of our Hope Heroes. A brain injury survivor for over forty years, Jeff has touched the lives of thousands through his prolific blogging, writing, and conference presentations that span many decades. It's not so much what happens to you, but what you do with your experience that really matters, as Jeff shows us all.

When **Mandi Seipel**'s son Colter fell from a second story window and sustained a brain injury, Mandi became driven to make sure that this same type of accident didn't happen to other families. Mandi continues to not only advocate window fall prevention but raises awareness on brain injuries and preventable accidents.

In August of 2012, **Norma Myers'** life forever changed. A horrific automobile accident took the life of her young son Aaron and left her other son Steven with a severe brain injury. In the years that have passed since this tragedy, Norma has become an ever-present voice within the brain injury community, a dedicated caregiver to Steven, and a prolific writer whose words have helped countess others worldwide.

Ted Stachulski used to work as an engineering and robotics technician and was skilled at multi-tasking and fast thinking. That all changed in 1999 when he was hit in his right temple at work by a piece of metal. This only added to the challenges he faced as a result of years of youth football, and the accompanying multiple concussions that come with the sport. Today, Ted is a tireless advocate helping fellow veterans, as well as a gifted writer, as his readers around the world can attest to.

To our 2019 Hope Heroes, on behalf of the worldwide community of brain injury survivors, family members, and caregivers, we thank you. Your actions, words, and deeds have touched and saved lives!

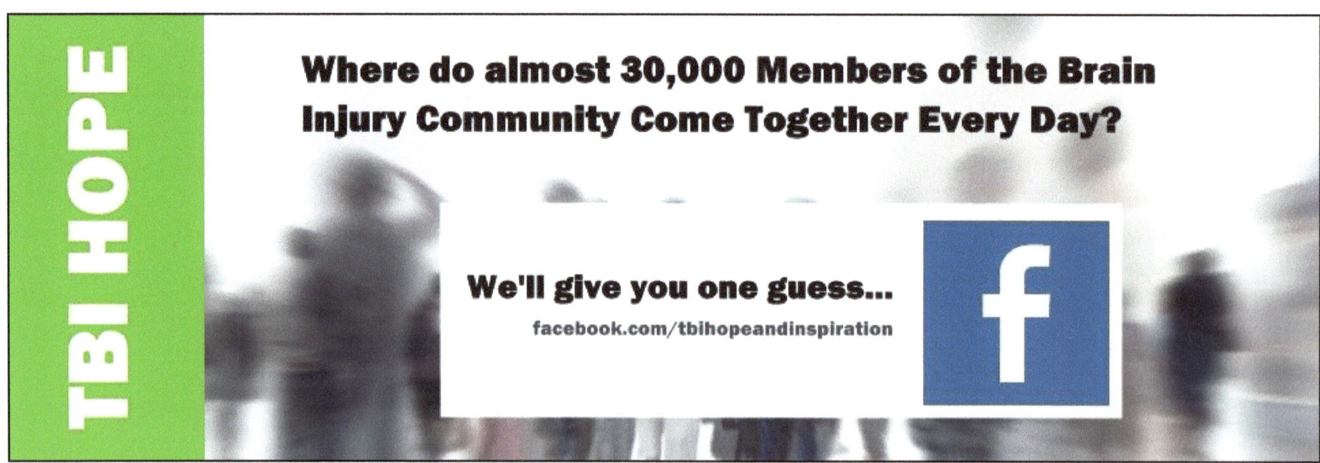

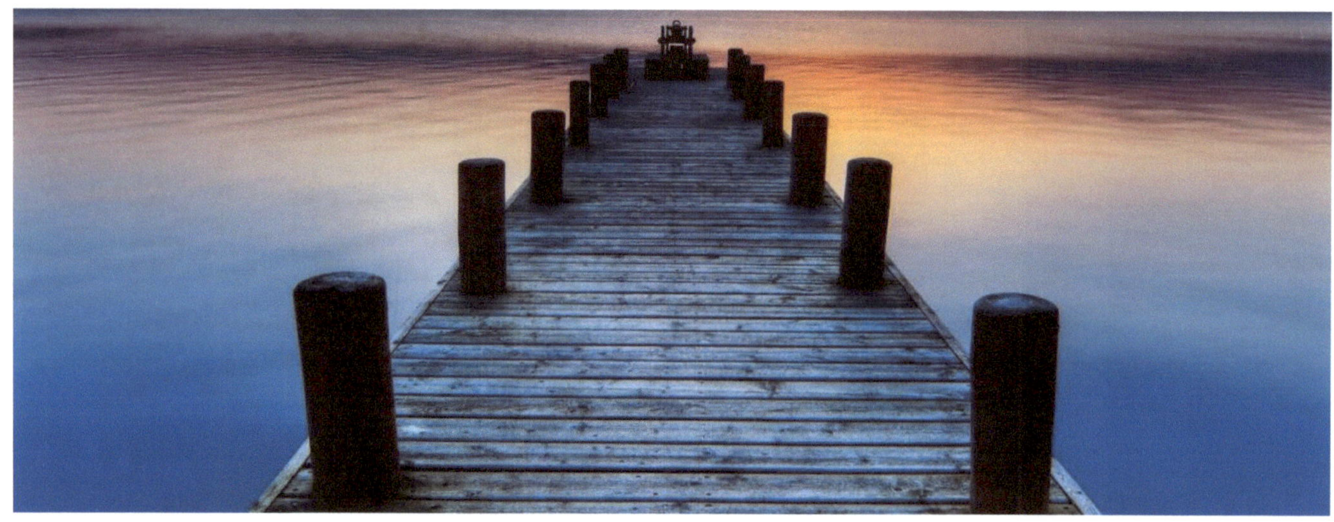

What Lies Within

By Rosemary Rawlins

The brain controls everything, so when a brain is injured, it feels as if everything's out of control, and there's nothing we humans love more than being in control.

I don't know what it's like to want to say one word and have another word come out of my mouth, or to try to walk, only to find my feet all tripped up, but I've witnessed the man I love most struggling to perform simple tasks, and I've felt out of control myself because I could not help him.

> "Many years have gone by now, and I've learned a good deal about resilience."

In the early days of caring for Hugh after his severe TBI, I'd feel a bit annoyed when people would say things like, "Take it one day at a time." I'd sometimes whisper in my mind, "How about YOU take it one day at a time, I'll go back to my old life, thank you!" Not nice thoughts, I know, but true. I wanted control. I wanted a problem I could fix.

Many years have gone by now, and I've learned a good deal about resilience. In a resilience study, Dr. Emilie Godwin reports that resilient individuals and families know how to "normalize crisis." The phrase sounds like an oxymoron to me. Normal and crisis don't belong together, like the words "awfully good" or "painfully lucky." But when I realized what she meant by this, it all made sense. Normalizing crisis simply means that people see their problems as something manageable, something they can handle. When we don't normalize crisis, we remain in crisis mode (one definition of crisis is "dangerous or worrying time") and we're stuck in a frame of mind that keeps us from moving forward. In short, we see our problems as hopeless.

Over the course of my entire experience as a caregiver I've learned this vital lesson: All of our problems have solutions. They are among us and within us.

We find solutions to our problems and even our crisis-like problems when we reach out to others, when we accept help, when we listen and follow sound advice. These are the solutions we find among us. When some problems prove too difficult to overcome, when they feel insurmountable and there seems to be no help available at all, the solution lies within us. We dig deep to find the fortitude, acceptance, and grace to move forward day by day until we eventually emerge from the fog as we draw strength from our personal faith and our human need to seek meaning from adversity.

Sometimes, the only answers to our problems lie within us. These answers may be hard to find, but they are worth seeking because they bring us peace. The first step is knowing they are there, inside us, waiting to be found.

> "We find solutions to our problems and even our crisis-like problems when we reach out to others, when we accept help, when we listen and follow sound advice."

Meet Rosemary Rawlins

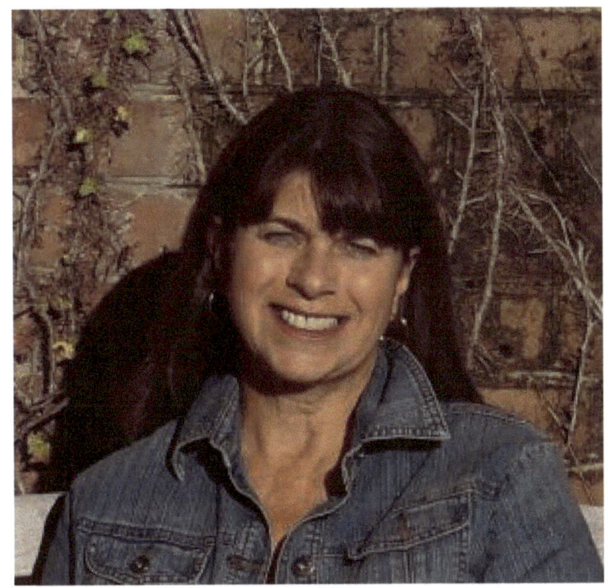

Rosemary Rawlins is the author of Learning by Accident: A Caregiver's True Story of Fear, Family, and Hope, an inspirational memoir about learning and growing through adversity.

When Rosemary's husband suffered a severe traumatic brain injury after a car hit him on his bike, she struggled for two years to bring him back home and back to himself, and when he was finally better, she fell apart. Rosemary has had many years of experience as a full-time caregiver for loved ones with brain injury, dementia, and COPD, and has a keen understanding of caregiver stress.

She is also Editor of BrainLine blogs and a national speaker on caregiving topics.

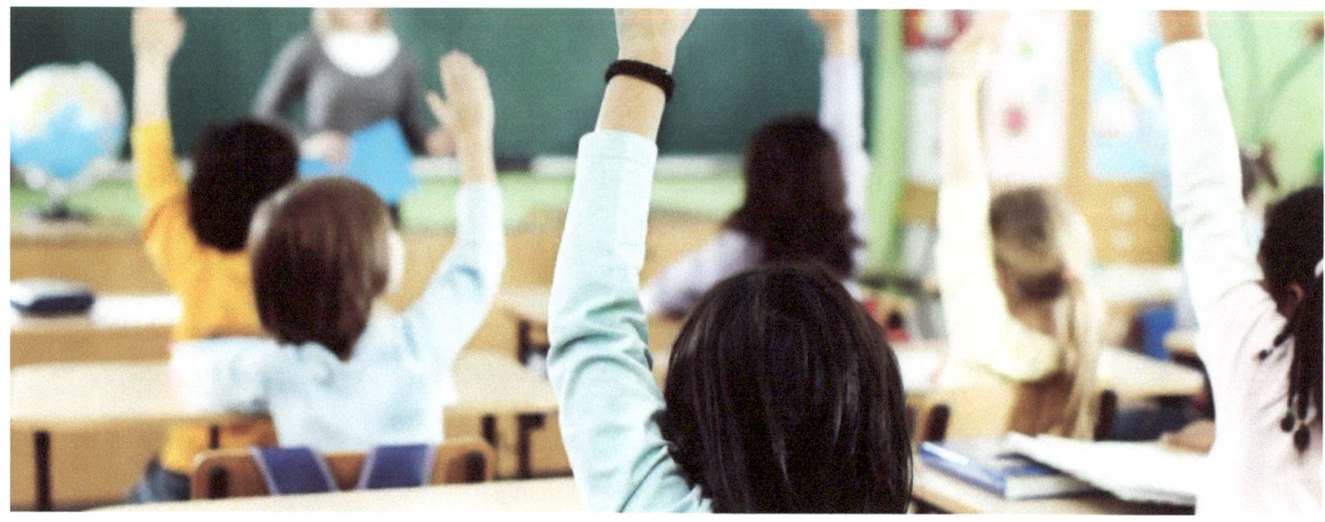

Making the Grade
By Nicole Bingaman

Close to a year and a half after my son's traumatic brain injury, we began working with a Neurological-psychologist. We found a terrific doctor, who seemed to grasp not only the medical side of brain injury, but also the emotional impact specifically relating to Taylor. Following a few sessions of becoming acquainted with Dr. Randy, cognitive testing was recommended. This would allow us to gain a better understanding of where Taylor's thinking processes were. A baseline could be established offering insight into a different aspect of the injury than that which was glaringly obvious.

I was still a fairly new student in the classroom of TBI, and was once again, not fully prepared for the lesson I was about to learn. Hours of testing took place and a few weeks later, we were called in to discuss the results. The fact that Taylor could undergo and complete the test process itself was an accomplishment, but sometimes even positive milestones feel painful.

> "I was still a fairly new student in the classroom of TBI, and was once again, not fully prepared for the lesson I was about to learn."

Up until this time in parenting I had been fortunate to have three sons who were healthy in mind and body. They had each successfully navigated their high school education, sports and extra-curricular activities. They were part of the National Honor Society, All-Star Sports Teams and took part in community service. Taylor even graduated first in his class at the technical school where he learned the skill of being an HVAC specialist.

As I sat with Dr. Randy that day listening to the results, I felt like the world was about to suck me in to another unexplored layer of sadness and shock. I could hear my heart beating, as my intuition warned me that something bad was about to happen. My body and mind prepared for the blow.

The doctor explained that Taylor was functioning at the level of someone who was around nine years old. He discussed the challenges in thought processing, understanding, word recognition, insight and an exhaustive list of things that represented more of what the injury had stripped away. I don't know what I came in expecting the results to convey, but it certainly was not that. I felt as if I was being punched in the gut. Ever aware that brain injury changes everything.

The strangest occurrence happened to me in those moments. I swallowed my tears, I took the deep breaths I had become accustomed to taking, I inwardly scolded myself for coming to the appointment alone and I heard again the silent scream that had become my friend in this classroom. That scream defined the emotion I could not let out, the parts of me that no one would ever see.

More of my son was gone that I realized. Then I saw something flash in front of my memory that has bothered me since that day. I saw the bumper sticker that said, "Proud Parent of An Honor Roll Student." The hurt and anger inside of me wondered what our bumper sticker would say, "My once strong, bright 22 year old is now functioning at the level of a nine year old." I was ashamed of my thoughts.

Questions like "Why did this happen to Taylor?" ran through my head, and the truth is they still do. But please understand this…I wish with all of my being that brain injury never happened to anyone…ever…again.

> **"My once strong, bright 22 year old is now functioning at the level of a nine year old."**

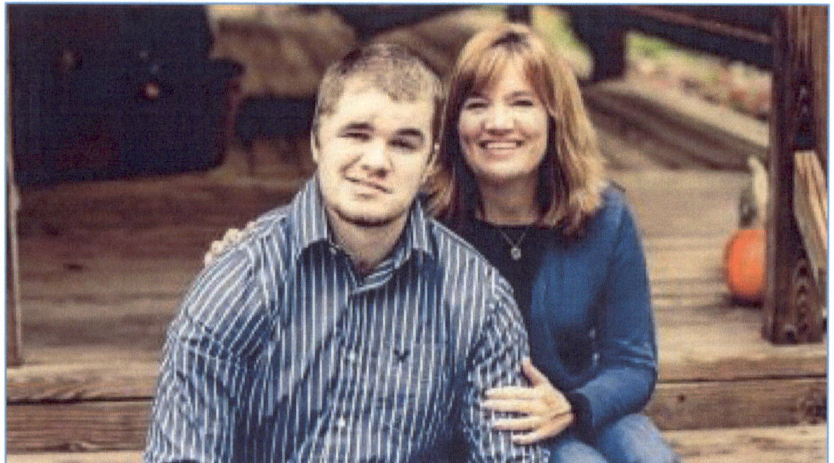

Since that time, Taylor has been retested. For round two's results, my husband and other sons came along. We sat together for the news. The test can only take place every two years, so they were spaced out for about that length of time. I came in to that meeting with fairly high hopes. Dr. Randy did not dive right in this time. Instead, he talked to each of us about what Taylor's injury meant in fairly concrete terms. We then discussed some ways that it affected our family and relationships. We were all uncomfortable in this room, with this psychologist, wondering how we ever got here. It has been said "the tension was so thick you could cut it with a knife," but what was thick that day, was pain.

On that day I learned a tremendous lesson. I learned that people are much more than their grades, their academic accomplishments or what club they belong to. Intellectually I knew that before, but now I knew it in my heart. There are beautiful souls, who are functioning at a level far less than their peers, who are more than exceptional and deserve recognition. Before then you may have heard me talk about GPA's, and various achievements, but that has become a part of life that I have let go. Those things matter, but they do not define a person.

Underneath all of the ink blots, timed sequences, and recognition of simple objects such as comb or toothbrush, was my son's mind. Taylor worked with his beautiful, broken brain, which was trudging through some thick mud to come back even the tiniest bit. And although the results were less than we had hoped, they were something to be proud of. In our society we are often impressed by the letters behind someone's name, PhD, MD, MA, and so on. The letters behind Taylor's name will always be, TBI survivor, and for that I will always be grateful.

Meet Nicole Bingaman

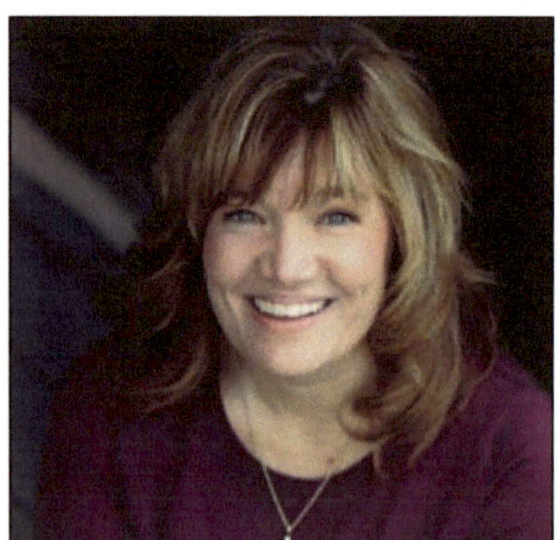

Nicole has worked in the human service field for over twenty years. Since Taylor's injury Nicole has become an advocate and spokesperson within the brain injury community. Nicole's book Falling Away From You was published and released in 2015. Nicole continues to share Taylor's journey on Facebook. Nicole firmly believes in the mantra "Love Wins."

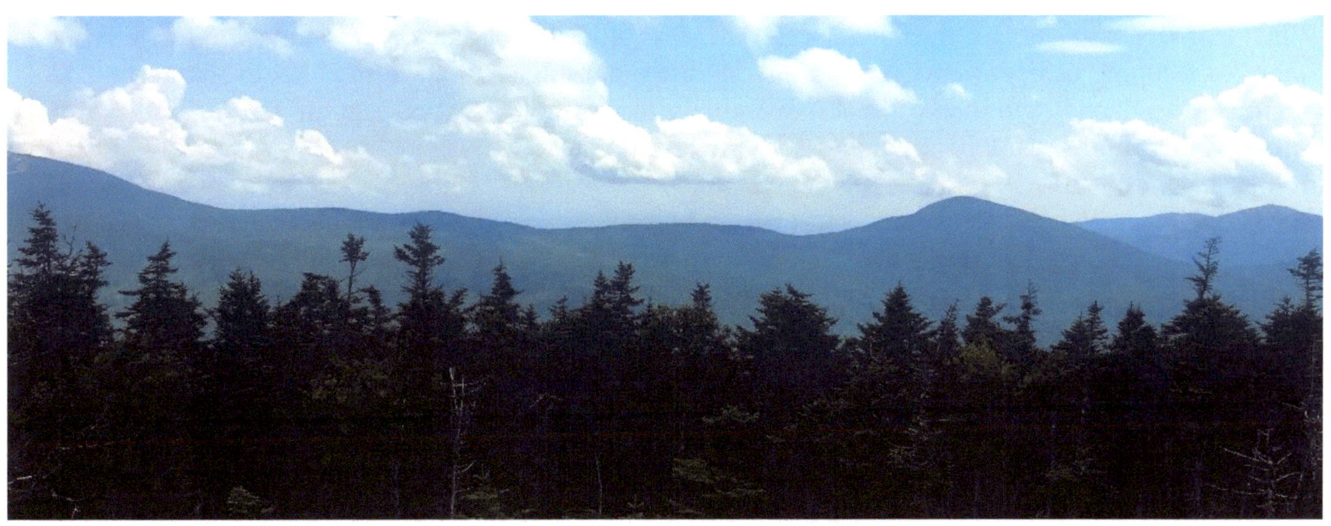

Overcoming Barriers
By Sarah Kilch Gaffney

I was fourteen or fifteen years old when I got my first concussion and nineteen when I received my last, amassing approximately eight in the intervening years. This occurred before we knew much about the cumulative nature of head injuries and before we paid much attention to them, and the last one was where they all caught up with me.

In my final college soccer game, I collided with a player from the opposing team. The details are fuzzy, but ultimately her knee connected directly under my chin. I was stunned and it took a few minutes to get me off the field. Sitting on the sideline, I took off my goalkeeper gloves and, realizing I had forgotten my mouth guard that day, palpated my jaw, grateful that my teeth were still intact.

> "When I brought up my continued symptoms, the athletic director told me that I did not need an evaluation and I certainly did not have a concussion."

My tongue swelled, and the student athletic trainer crushed up something so that I could swallow it. The next day, I was exhausted and in pain. My parents, both former EMTs, wanted me to be evaluated. When I brought up my continued symptoms, the athletic director told me that I did not need an evaluation and I certainly did not have a concussion because "he saw concussions every day in football."

When I finally saw a doctor over a week later, I was told I had classic concussion symptoms. After weeks of sleeping nearly twenty hours a day, taking incompletes in all of my classes that term, and months of headaches and medications, I eventually recovered. I stopped playing soccer and swore off activities that might easily result in another knock to the head.

The following summer, I decided to serve as an AmeriCorps volunteer on a backcountry trail crew in the Maine wilderness. There, on a mountain on the Appalachian Trail, I met Steve, a tall, lanky fellow from northern Vermont. Less than two years later, on a bright October day, Steve and I were married on that same mountain.

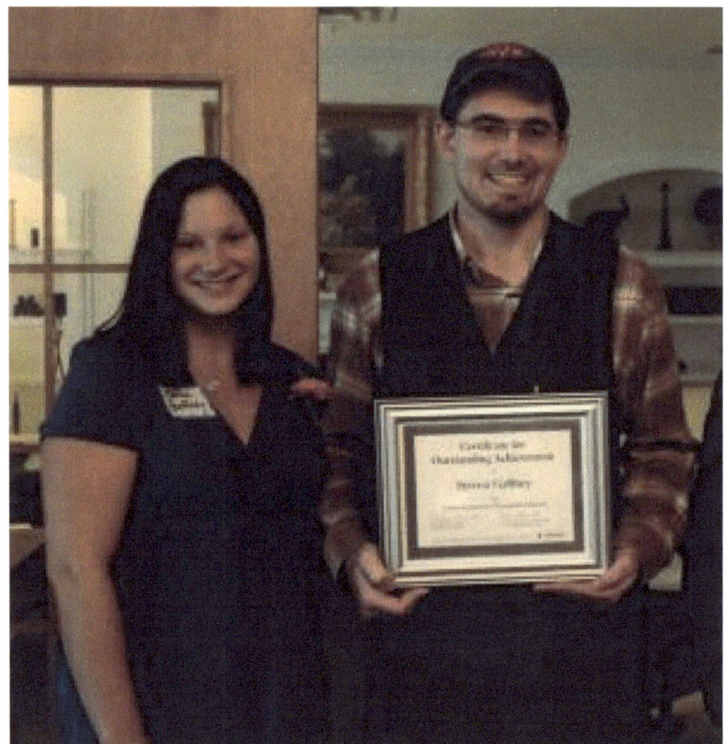

Shortly after our third wedding anniversary, Steve and I arrived back at our car after a weekend hike, and he couldn't speak. First there was silence, then gibberish, then real words but in no logical order, then it was as if nothing at all had happened. He was completely back to himself and assured me he was fine.

The following day, Steve was diagnosed with a massive brain tumor. He was 27 years old.

Steve was a champion of patience and humor, attributes that had served him well in his work teaching others how to build trails, and he held onto his good nature and easy-going attitude as we faced an uncertain future.

He joked, laughed, and smiled his way through two awake brain surgeries, radiation, multiple chemotherapies, and proton beam radiation. I can't count the number of times we walked down the halls of his cancer center hand in hand with me in tears and him telling me it was going to be okay.

When he awoke from the first brain surgery with cognitive and speech challenges, Steve dove head first into speech therapy, earning himself an *"Overcoming Barriers"* award from our local hospital. When the radiation therapy left him permanently disabled, he maintained his positive outlook. When he became homebound during the last few months of his life, he was still able to smile – a fact for which I will always be extremely grateful and in absolute awe of.

Shortly after his diagnosis, Steve's oncologist had revealed to us that his tumor would eventually be terminal, and we tried our best to live our life while carrying that knowledge. Along the way, our daughter was born, and Steve loved her with absolutely everything he had.

Steve's doctors never talked about brain injuries. Though, of course, that is what he was experiencing, over and over again. His oncologist was concerned with the efficacy of chemotherapy, his neurosurgeon with the delicate balance of cutting too much versus too little, his neurologist with controlling his seizures. And, so, no one talked about brain injuries, or what to expect, or where to seek help, support, or information. We didn't even talk to a social worker until the week before Steve started hospice.

Until the last couple weeks of his life, Steve had little pain. His fatigue, however, was immense and unrelenting. Everything made him tired and each new treatment increased the weight of that burden, building over the years.

As treatments failed and his tumor progressed, Steve slowly lost cognitive and physical function. Eventually, he could no longer walk, no longer leave the house, and then no longer leave the hospital bed that we had squeezed into our bedroom.

Steve died at home two months shy of his 32nd birthday, four and a half years after his diagnosis. I found myself reeling, widowed with a toddler, and with no idea what to do or how to make my way through life now that Steve was no longer by my side.

When Steve became disabled, I had started working towards nursing school. We had both continued to work in the conservation field after we met, but I felt that I now needed a different career to support our family. I fought hard to follow through with that decision, juggling Steve's treatments and care with raising our daughter, work, school, and managing a house.

I left nursing school to take care of Steve during the last months of his life, and returned after he died, but despite my 4.0 GPA and outward success, I was miserable and it became clear that it was no longer where I needed to be. At the time, it seemed hard to believe that there would ever be another right path, but I desperately needed a change and a break.

I didn't take much of a break, but I did find the change that I needed. A little over a year after Steve's death and just over a month after I left nursing school, I accepted a position as the Program Coordinator for the Brain Injury Association of America's Maine Chapter. It's a dream job, and I still sometimes pinch myself to make sure it's real.

Now, I get to spend my days increasing awareness about brain injury, helping survivors and families get the resources and support that they need, and being an important voice for those with brain injury in Maine. I get to provide the support that didn't exist when Steve was sick, and I get to make sure survivors and families aren't without somewhere to turn when they have questions or need help. I cannot think of a better way to honor Steve's memory and I am grateful for the opportunity every day.

Meet Sarah Kilch Gaffney

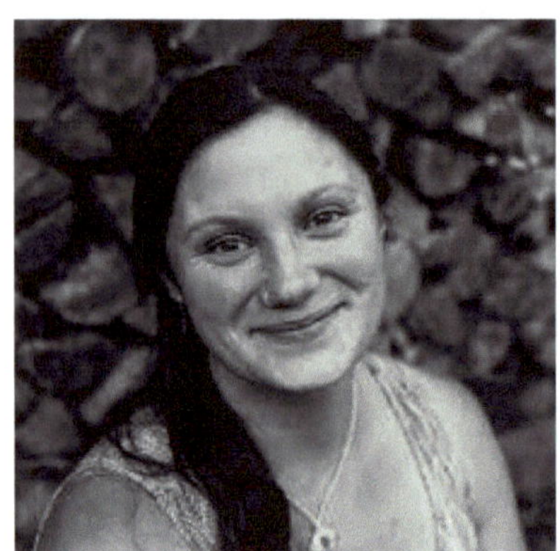

Sarah Kilch Gaffney is a writer, brain injury advocate, and homemade caramel aficionado. You can visit BIAA-ME's website at www.biausa.org/maine and you can find her writing at www.sarahkilchgaffney.com.

Living With Hope

By Patrick Brigham

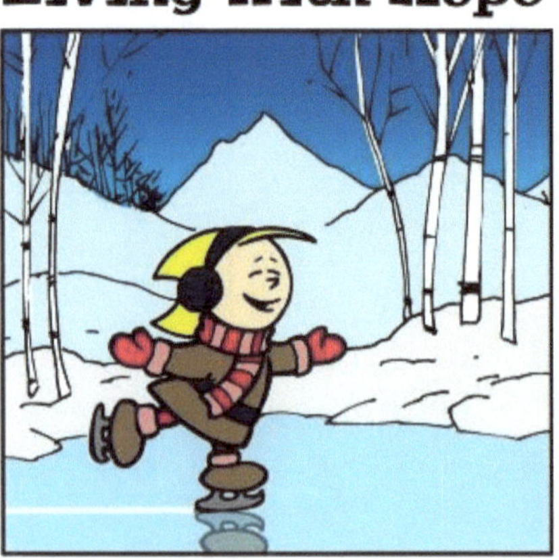

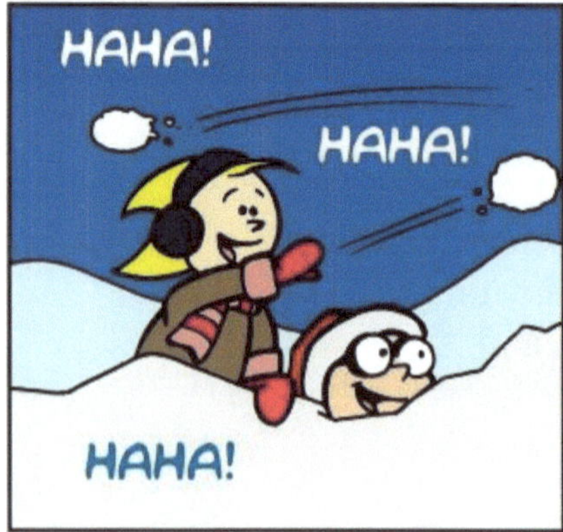

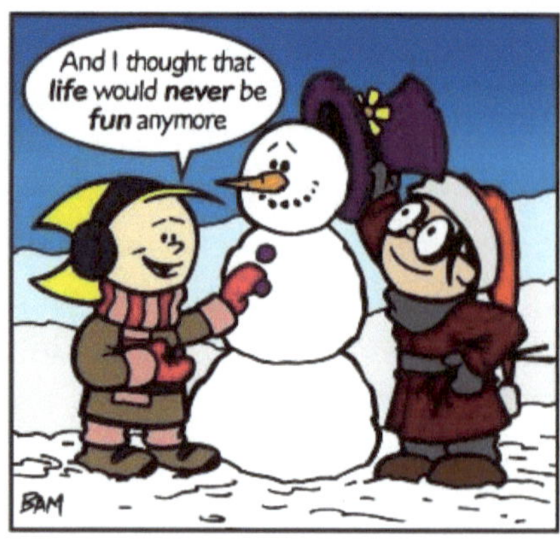

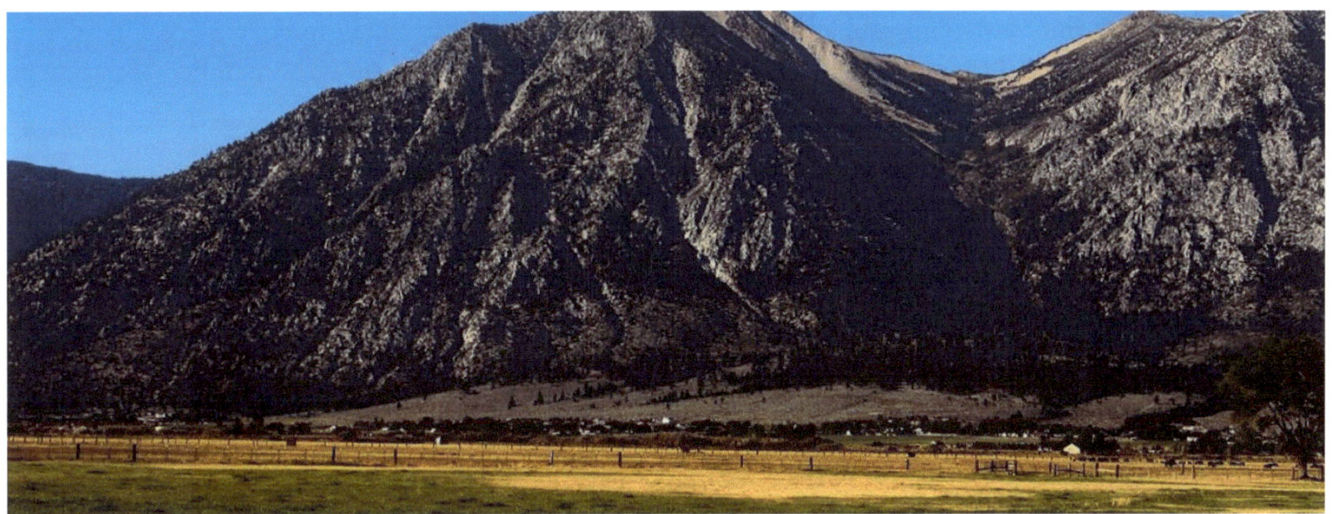

Because I Can!

By Rosalie Johnson

When I go to Florida in my motorhome, it's a fresh start. Each day is planned and planned again, well in advance, using the strategies I learned while recovering from a Traumatic Brain Injury.

On the road, I can only move forward. I can still remember my other life: work, volunteer, play, maintain a home and still have plenty of time to spend with my husband Randy, family, and friends.

> "Like most survivors, I remember when that world crashed – December 8, 2001."

Like most survivors, I remember when that world crashed – December 8, 2001. In my new reality, I feel as if I am a child's toy top spinning so fast that the centrifugal force is randomly spewing away my thoughts and plans to be productive. Some days the top slows down, and on others, it rotates so quickly that it is all I can do just to hang on and ride.

Travel gives me back control. With my itinerary plan and the larders stocked, Randy tries to start the trip with me. We head south in the late winter. Each day we drive 250-300 miles easing into a routine and trying to miss any snowstorm in the forecast. Arriving at an RV campground, we level the motorhome, extend the slides, and connect the water and sewer.

Next, I walk the "Road Warrior" – my old Yorkie, Lilly. Then there is dinner to prepare, clean up, and finally sleep. The next morning the routine is reversed. Any items we used must be stowed, as they become projectiles while traveling. At some airport along the route, I usually have to drop

Randy off to fly home, so he can return to work. You should see some of the looks we get when driving our motorhome through the departure area of an airport! Being a pilot, he will be able to meet me at future destinations down the road.

I spend a week here or two weeks there, eventually making it all the way to Key West. Every day is planned, such as stopping for gas or groceries along the way, because once the RV is parked and set up, I can't just drive to any store. I get around on my bicycle for planned adventures. I am very fortunate to have family and friends join me along the way. I love the company for exploring new areas but there is one stipulation: they have to be ready to bicycle or walk everywhere. Just ask my friend, Anne, about her "Vacation Boot Camp!" I have baskets and coolers to attach to our bicycles, along with a cart to carry groceries, laundry, or beach chairs.

When traveling alone, I am rarely lonely. Walking Lilly, I meet many other dogs. Each evening finds most campers at the waterfront to marvel at the beauty of the sunset. More bonds form. The people I encounter are from all over the world, and all share the same bond: "Wanderlust." In meeting so many interesting folks, the number of Traumatic Brain Injury and Stroke survivors is astounding.

With one particular couple, the wife suffered a stroke some years ago. Each evening her husband bundles her up and helps her into their golf cart, then drives to the waterfront to watch the sunset. Due to the severity of her aphasia, she is only able to speak three words. She will take each person's hand, place it on her heart, look deeply into their eyes and say "I love you, I LOVE YOU!" Is there any better way to share a sunset? Along the way, I'm invited to join other RV'ers for potluck dinners, Yoga, airplane rides, museum tours, and much, much more. The people I have the pleasure to meet share so much of their lives with me. They are like little gifts. Each day I learn something new: the name of a flower or tree, or the mating habits of dolphins or alligators.

When learning that I am a Traumatic Brain Injury survivor, many other travelers will ask me how I can drive the RV and do all of the set up mostly alone. I respond, "Because I can!"

Meet Rosalie Johnson

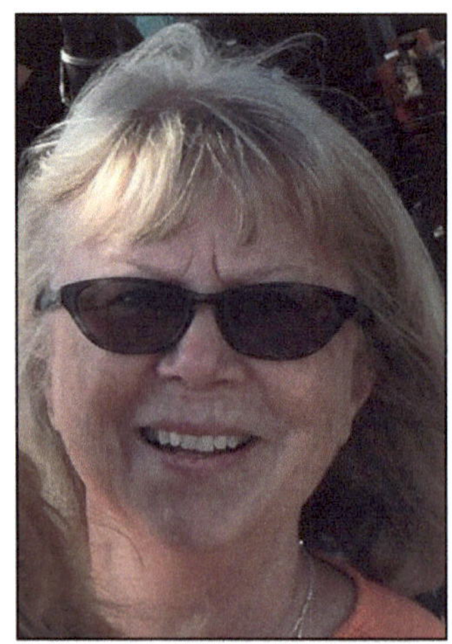

Before her Traumatic Brain Injury, Rosalie Johnson was a Registered Nurse and loved volunteering for various non-profit organizations. She was able to travel, and live and work throughout the country with her husband, Randy and their ever-changing family of dogs.

These days Rosalie can be found running the Seacoast Brain Injury Support Group and volunteering at Krempels Center in Portsmouth, New Hampshire. She is a seven-year Board Member for the Brain Injury Association of New Hampshire, author of "Meet the Artist" article printed quarterly in HEADWAY Newsletter published by BIANH.

Finding Senior Housing can be complex, but it doesn't have to be.

Call A Place for Mom. Our Advisors are trusted, local experts who can help you understand your options. Since 2000, we've helped over one million families find senior living solutions that meet their unique needs.

"You can trust **A Place for Mom** to help you."

– Joan Lunden

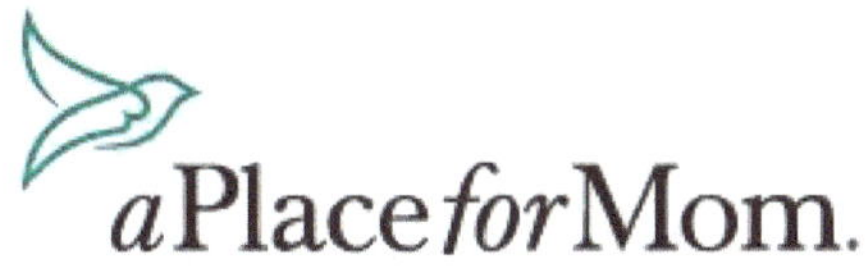

A Free Service for Families.

Call: (844) 578-9504

A Place for Mom is the nation's largest senior living referral information service. We do not own, operate, endorse or recommend any senior living community. We are paid by partner communities, so our services are completely free to families.

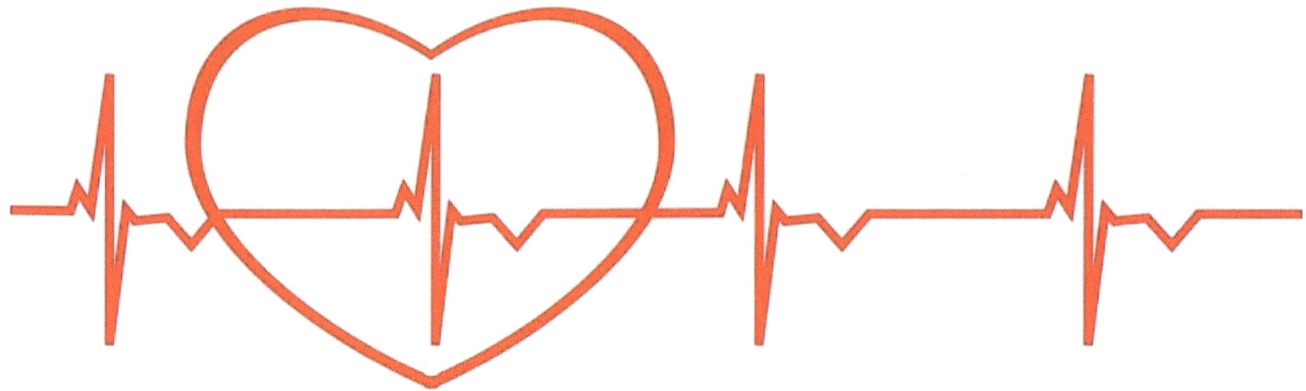

Healing Your Heart After Brain Injury

By Barbara J. Webster

Winter can be a tough season for anyone, but it can be exceptionally difficult for a brain injury survivor. On top of struggling with the winter weather, limiting outdoor activities due to the cold temperatures or slippery surfaces and the typical "winter blues," brain injury survivors are often struggling with a fundamental Life Crisis: who am I and what is my value if I can't do what I used to do, if my friends aren't my friends anymore and I'm a problem for my family?

Something essential that I learned and wish I'd known during my journey is that there is usually a grieving process associated with healing from a brain injury. I learned that there are common stages associated with the grieving process: denial, anger, bargaining, depression & acceptance. I also learned that processing grief is not a straightforward path, that one typically moves back and forth in the different stages

> "There is usually a grieving process associated with healing from a brain injury."

and that is "normal." I learned that in order to heal and be able to move forward, it is necessary to recognize your feelings, acknowledge the losses, allow yourself to feel the feelings and mourn the losses.

The devastating losses brain injury survivors experience are far-reaching. On top of struggling with physical injuries and cognitive deficits, there are usually secondary losses as well: income, jobs, social networks, friends, even family and homes. Survivors often lose much of their life that took years, sometimes many decades, to build.

Needless to say, the changes and losses I experienced had a profound effect on me and on my Being. I had lost my self-confidence and my "sense of self." I was becoming more and more depressed.

Something else to consider is that your family and friends may be grieving too. When you think about it, they have lost the person you used to be and the role you used to play in their lives as well.

Getting in touch with my spiritual guides was instrumental in helping me move through the grieving process and heal my heart. I needed to hear, to be re-taught, that I had value in my Being, not just in my doing. Being part of a support group for brain injury survivors let me know I was not alone in my struggle. Many find it necessary to seek professional help to help them cope with and navigate this complex process.

One of the keys for me was to forgive myself; forgive myself for not being able to do what I used to be able to do; forgive myself for being human. I also needed to forgive others for their shortcomings, for being human. Ignoring your feelings will hold you back. Your grief and whatever way it manifests in your life will create stress and inhibit your rehabilitation process overall. Our brains work best when we feel well, physically and emotionally.

"We are human 'beings', not human 'doings.'" ~Bernie Siegel

"We are human 'beings', not human 'thinkings.'" ~ Deepak Chopra

Strategies that can be helpful:

♥ Keep a Grateful Journal, writing down 3 things every day that were successful, an improvement, or made you smile.

♥ Arrange regular get-togethers with friends, even if just to chat on the phone or to meet for a cup of coffee or tea.

♥ Spend some time on a hobby.

♥ Practice random acts of kindness.

♥ Volunteer.

♥ Get some physical exercise, every day.

♥ Go outdoors; soak up some fresh air, sunshine and vitamin D.

♥ Sign up for a class, anything that interests you.

♥ Think about what is most important to you and how you can bring more of it into your life.

♥ Keep your perspective, refer to your calendar and journals to look back and note improvements. Celebrate what you can do now that you couldn't do six months or a year ago.

♥ Remember that you are still the same unique and valuable person inside, with the same loves that you had before your injury. No one and no injury can take that away from you.

Depression, like winter, is usually temporary, but if you feel like you are losing hope, please seek professional help.

Meet Barbara J. Wester

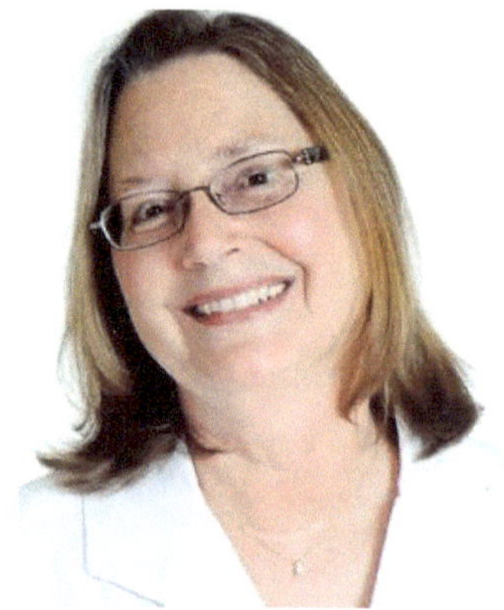

Barbara J. Webster is author of Lost and Found, A Survivors Guide for Reconstructing Life after a Brain Injury, Lash & Assoc. Publishing and a contributor to Chicken Soup for the Traumatic Brain Injury Survivor's Soul.

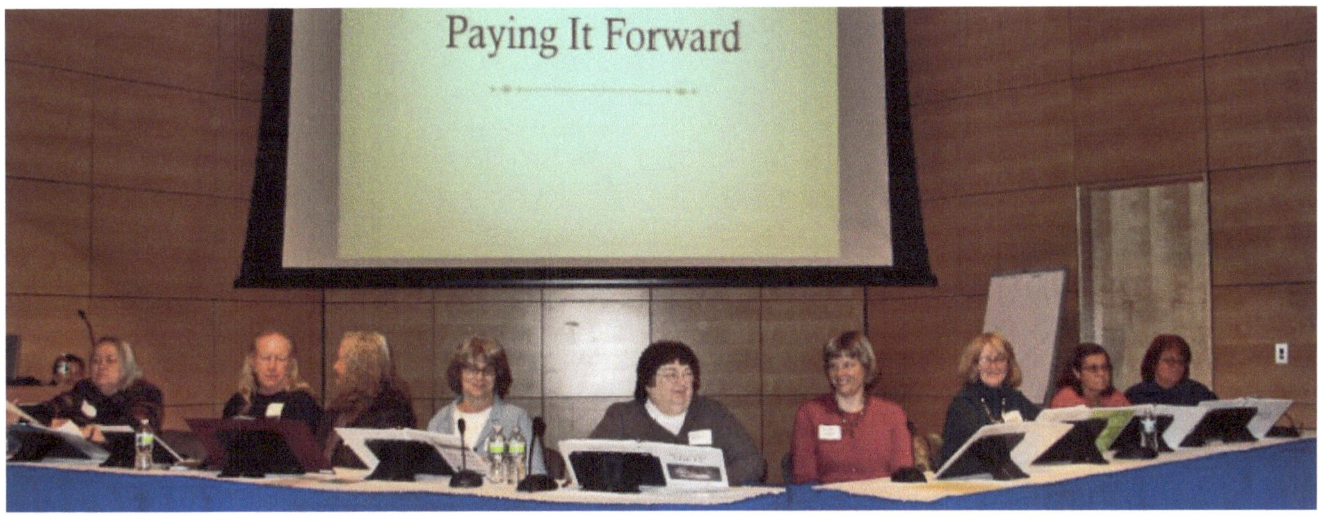

Pearls of Wisdom

Compiled by Carole Starr

Bev Bryant (1939-2014), pictured above in the middle, was an author, national speaker and co-founder of Brain Injury Voices. In her memory, Voices members extracted these 'pearls of wisdom' from her books and speeches…

Aim High
"I have learned that if we can keep our life full of optimism and positive thinking, that we can conquer anything that happens to us and look forward to the next challenge with confidence and determination."

Learn from Failure
I have the right to fail. I do not plan to, but I have that right. No one, absolutely no one, will ever take that right away from me. It is from that failure that I will move onward. It is from that failure that I will grow. It is from those failures that I will dare to be silent no more. It is from those failures that I will forge my excellence. There is no loss in failing because I am making the attempt to succeed and face the challenge. The only real failure is never trying in the first place.

Live in the Present
We cannot compare the past with the present, then and now. We have to live for today and plan for tomorrow.

Find the Humor

Humor is about a state of being. It's about attitudes, optimism, and being happy. It's about being happy INSIDE one's self. It's about seeing things and events in a different light and from a different perspective. As a result of this new vantage point, you may also see new ways to deal with the problems…We must be able to find humor even in our failures…. Do we look at them as walls and obstacles? Or can we accept those failures as building blocks or stepping-stones.

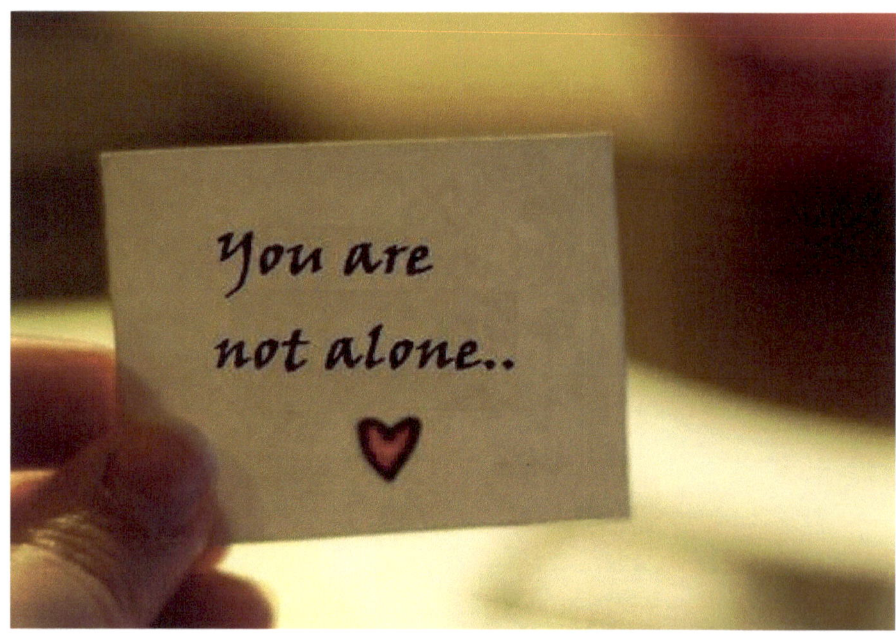

Take Steps to Heal

Healing takes place from the inside out. Healing involves the struggle to rebuild relationships with family, friends and colleagues. Healing is recognizing the grieving process and coming to grips with our remaining strengths, asking for accommodations, using strategies, compensating for weaknesses and believing in ourselves.

Find the Help you Need

Because of our brain injuries, we are forced to rebuild our flight path and rise up alone. We need professionals to help us rebuild the runway. The trek itself, in search of wings, can only be taken by the survivor… I need the strength of my friends and colleagues, certainly not their sympathy.

Meet Carole Starr

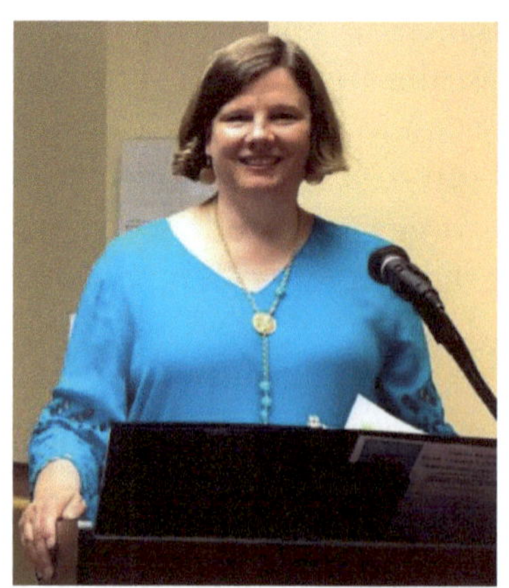

Carole Starr sustained a brain injury in a car accident in 1999. She's now an inspiring keynote speaker, the author of the book To Root & To Rise: Accepting Brain Injury, and the leader of Brain Injury Voices, an award-winning survivor education, advocacy and peer mentoring group in Maine.

To contact Carole, watch videos of her speeches or read an excerpt from her book, please visit StarrSpeakerAuthor.com.

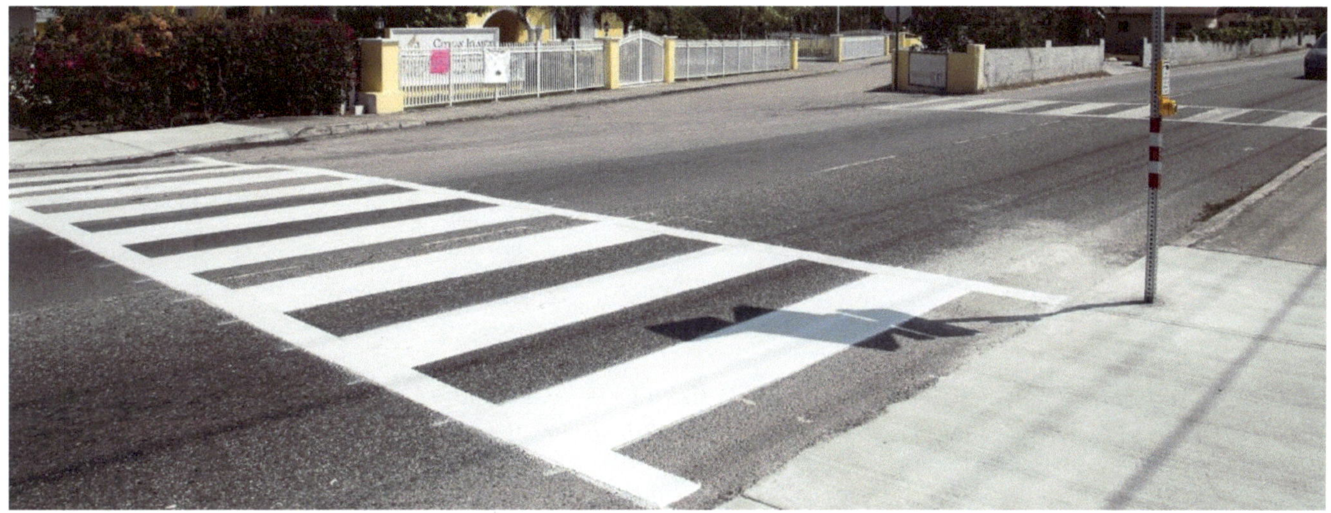

I Stumbled but Did Not Fall

By Donna Figurski

Recently, as I got out of my car, I stumbled on the curb. Somehow in the darkness, I did not see it. Though the event took less than a second, one thought ran through my head. It was not, "Oh, no! I am going to break a bone or scrape my knee." It was not, "What a klutz! I'll ruin my clothes." And it was not about how embarrassed I would be. All of those possibilities probably would have been my first thoughts before brain injury entered my life in 2005 when my husband had a traumatic brain injury.

Now my mind is only a thought away from brain injury. So, as I tripped and stumbled, but did not fall, I thought, "Please don't let me hit my head." I didn't care how silly I looked or about my clothes being ripped or about getting any broken bones (they would heal). I was concerned about getting a brain injury.

> "I worried about how a brain injury could change my life forever."

I worried about how a brain injury could change my life forever. I worried that if I were hurt, I could not sufficiently care for my husband, who needs my daily attention. Yes, those thoughts raced through my head in that fleeting second.

It only takes a second for a brain injury to occur. Most brain injuries occur because of an accident. Though we may be aware of the possibility of accidents, we cannot avoid all of them. Fortunately, my accident was avoided – just barely. I can only hope that my potential accidents will be few and far apart in the future. I hope yours will be too.

Meet Donna Figurski

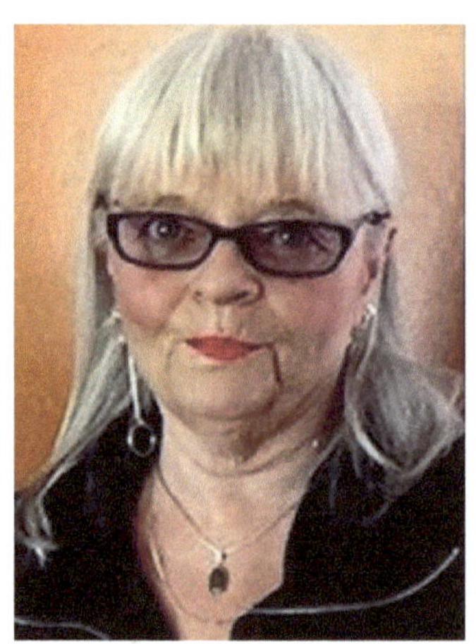

Donna Figurski, whose life revolves around traumatic brain injury (TBI), is a wife, mother, granny, teacher, playwright, actor, director, picture-book reviewer, radio host, speaker, photographer, and writer.

As a brain injury advocate, Donna has published articles in many brain-injury-related magazines on the web; has written chapters included in two books; writes a blog called "Surviving Traumatic Brain Injury"; is host of her international radio show, "Another Fork in the Road," online on the Brain Injury Radio Network, and is a speaker concerned with survivors of brain injury and their caregivers.

HOPE Magazine Featured Title

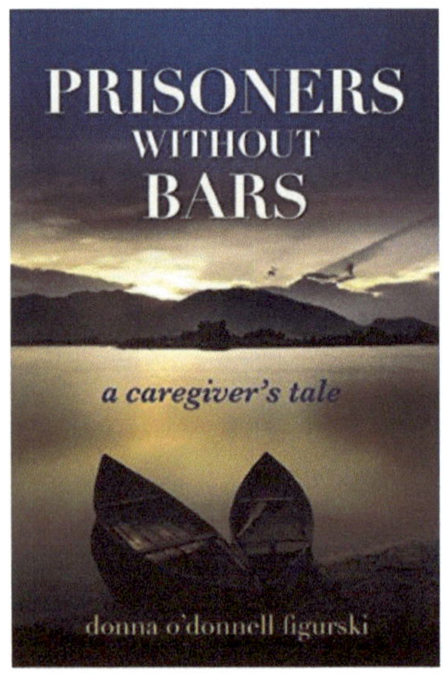

Prisoners Without Bars: A Caregiver's Tale

**This heart-wrenching and triumphant love story
is a tale of advocacy and caregiving.**

Available in Print & eBook

Order Your Copy Today!

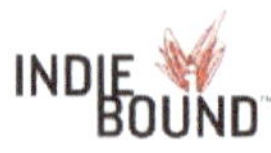

amazon　　BARNES&NOBLE　　INDIE BOUND

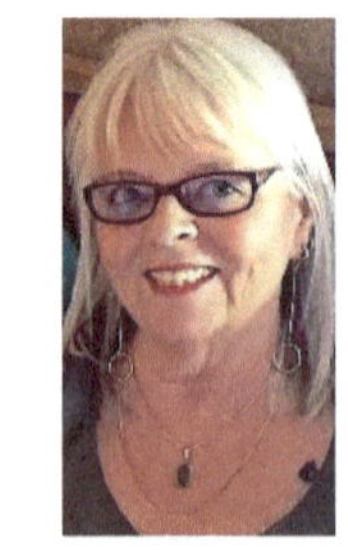

Donna O'Donnell Figurski
Author, Caregiver, Speaker, Radio Host
www.donnafigurski.com

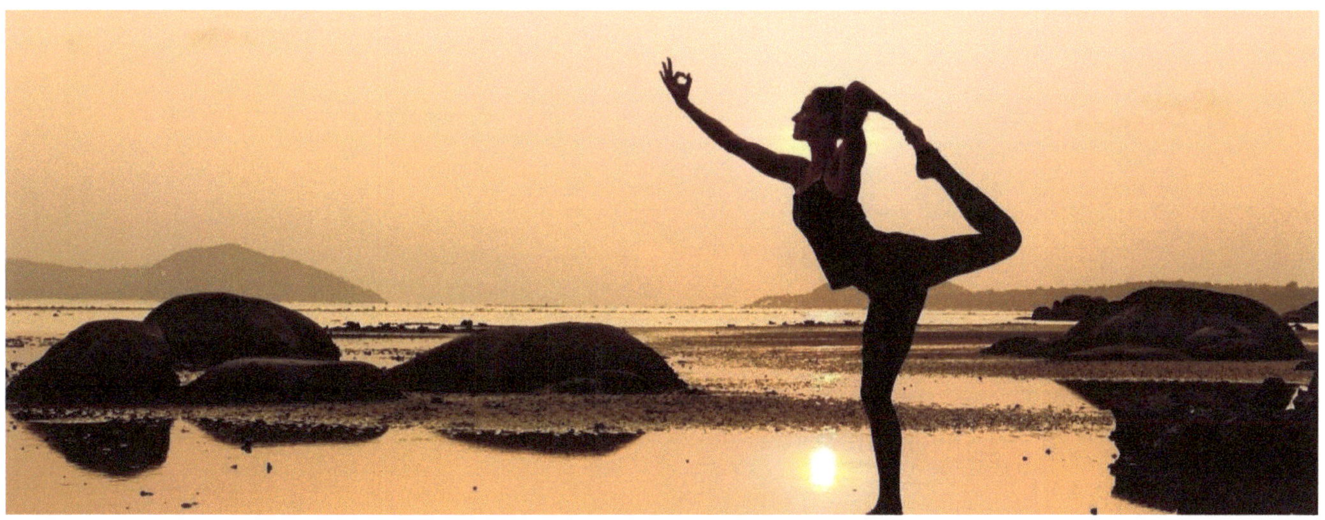

How Yoga Helped Me

By Amy Zellmer

On a cold February morning, my life changed forever. Walking down the driveway of my building, I slipped on a patch of sheer ice. My feet went straight up, and I landed with my head taking the full impact, briefly knocking me unconscious.

When I started to get up, I knew I wasn't okay. I had an excruciating pain in my skull where my head hit, and I was seeing whirly, bright lights out of my left eye.

A visit to the doctor confirmed I had a severe concussion, major whiplash, C4/5 damage, a dislocated sternum, and multiple torn muscles. I had no idea the road to recovery I would face, and how drastically my life had just changed.

> "I felt like I would never find any relief, and worried that the TBI would leave me permanently impaired."

I had been doing yoga since college because it brought me balance and peace and was an instant stress reliever for me. With all of my physical injuries added to my traumatic brain injury (TBI), I could no longer do yoga.

After months of vertigo, dizziness and balance issues, cognitive problems, short-term memory loss, and the pain of my physical injuries, I was at the end of my rope. I felt like I would never find any relief, and worried that the TBI would leave me permanently impaired and unable to ever do physical exercise again.

I consulted with a neurologist, chiropractic neurologist, as well as the National Dizzy and Balance Center. I was encouraged to attempt some physical movement, as it would eventually help my body work out its kinks and stabilize my balance issues. It seemed counter intuitive at the time; however, I was desperate to have some sense of normalcy and routine in my life.

About fifteen months after my accident, I took private lessons with my yoga instructor in an attempt to find poses I could do—poses that wouldn't trigger my vertigo or cause tension in my neck or sternum/clavicle area.

My instructor taught me how to use a chair or wall to support myself in standing poses so I didn't feel like I was going to fall. We found several poses I could do with modifications that didn't cause any problems or flare ups, including: Tree, Mountain, Cat/Cow, Puppy Dog, Forward Bend, and Seated Spine Twist.

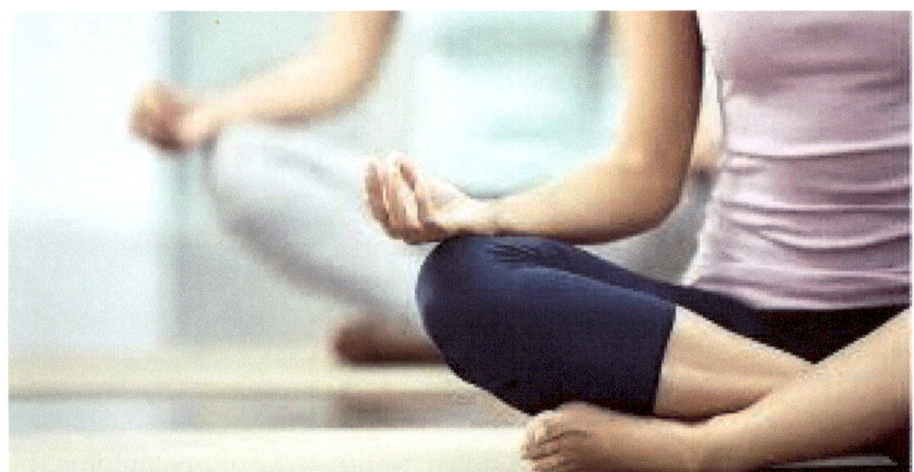

Within about six weeks of doing these poses every day for 10 minutes, I gradually added Down Dog, Plank, and Warrior for a breath. My vertigo and dizzy issues seemed to almost completely subside, and my balance was coming back closer to what it was pre-accident. Now with modifications I can do many of the poses I used to do. I still can't do any back bends or tip my head backwards, but I am on an amazing road to recovery, thanks to yoga.

I urge anyone with a TBI or other injury to try to incorporate yoga into your daily routine. If you think, "I'm not flexible, I can't do yoga," you are absolutely wrong!

If I can do this, *I know you can too!*

1. Listen to your body.
Don't do anything that hurts or causes you pain. Mild discomfort is to be expected if you haven't stretched your body in a while, however, if it actually hurts, listen to your body. Don't do that particular pose or modify it to fit what your body is capable of. If a pose triggers vertigo, try modifying it so that your head doesn't have to move, or else move on to a different pose.

2. Connect your breath.
Oxygen is critical for brain health, and yoga helps you connect your breath to your movements. Take strong, deep inhalations, and allow the out-breath to help you get deeper into the pose and deeper into the now ~ releasing all negative thoughts and emotions.

3. Modify poses.

In the beginning I could only do 5 simple, basic, stretching poses. I had to use a chair or wall to hold onto for balance. I couldn't do any poses that required my head forward or backward. Don't feel obligated to do every pose in a series, do what you can do and go at your own pace. Yoga is an individual "sport" and there is no one to impress other than yourself.

4. Believe in yourself.

I know it's a challenge when you haven't been able to do physical exercise in months, but I finally took the plunge and I know you can too! Yoga has SO many health benefits, and I truly believe in you and your ability to get moving and start feeling better. Let go of the resistance that is holding you back and allow yourself to move forward in your recovery! Your mind, body, and spirit will thank you!

Meet Amy Zellmer

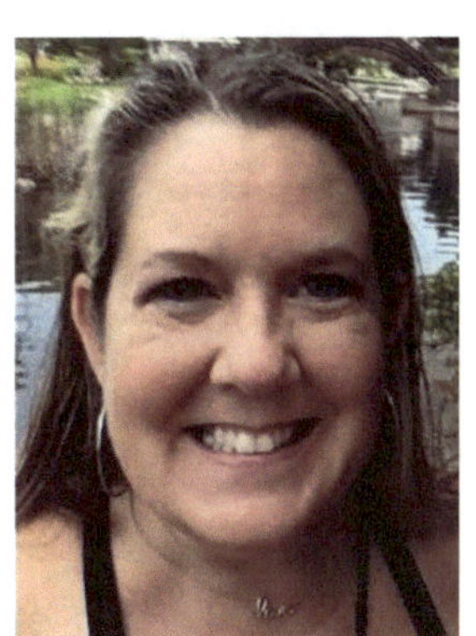

Amy Zellmer is a professional photographer and author located in Saint Paul, MN. She suffered a traumatic brain injury in February 2014, and is currently advocating to raise awareness about the severity of concussions and TBI. She released her first book "Life With a Traumatic Brain Injury: Finding the Road Back to Normal," in 2015.

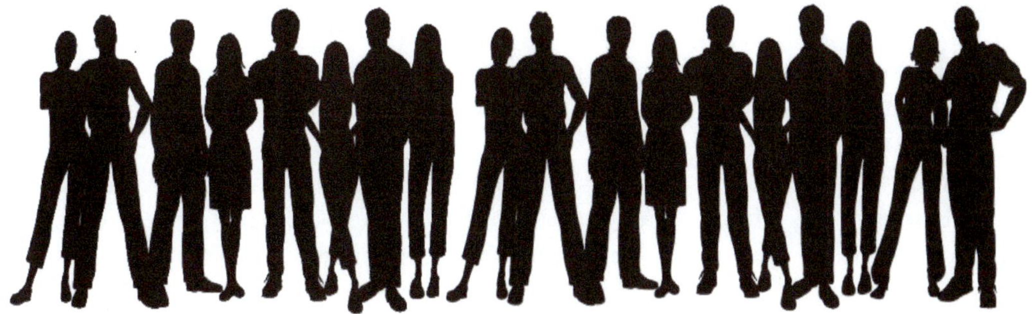

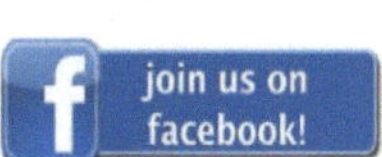

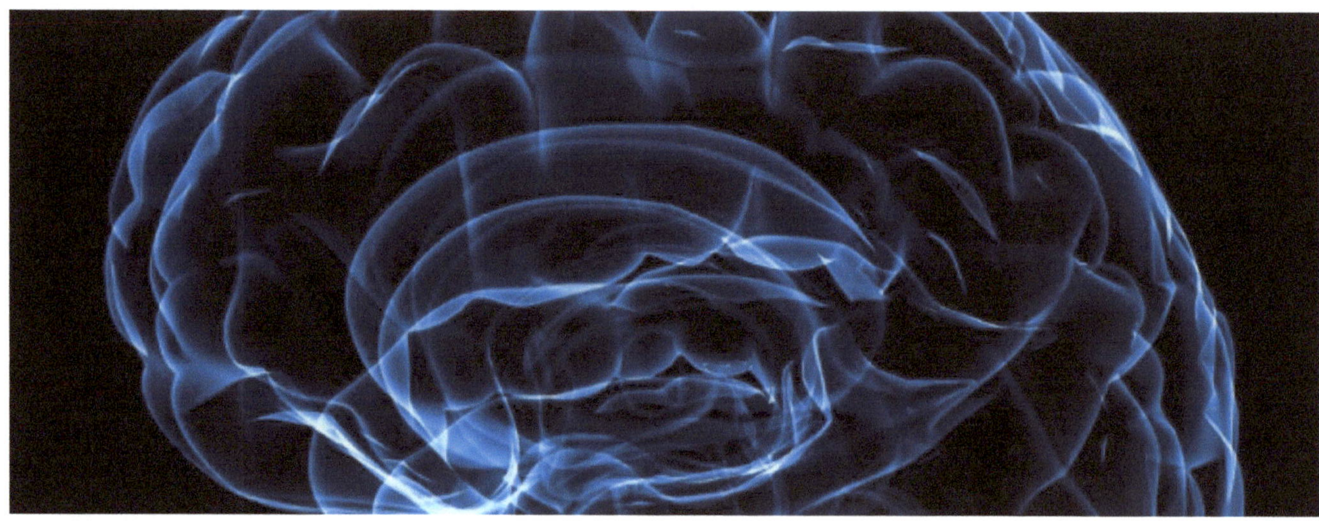

The Day I Broke my Brain
By Darron Eastwell

I have always loved mountain biking. There is something indescribably wonderful about being out on the trails. Fully immersed in nature you never know what you are going to see, and what you'll experience. Every ride is a completely unique experience.

In late May of 2015, I planned on a day of mountain bike riding at Tewantin National Park. Located on the Sunshine Coast in Queensland, Australia, Tewantin is a mountain biker's dream. The terrain is varied, with some very aggressive climbs.

> "Little did I know that my life, and the lives of those who love me, would be drastically changed forever."

It was a perfect day for riding. But, unfortunately, fate had other plans for me that day.

My GPS speedometer indicated that I had been riding for a couple of hours. As I have no memories from that day, I can only rely on the data. My pace was slow and easy as I rode. The hills were steep and I was enjoying my ride. The speedometer data show an abrupt jump in my speed up to almost 60km per hour (almost 40 MPH). It was clear that I had entered into a steep downhill descent.

This was to be the last cycling descent of my past life.

The day that started so sunny and full of bright promise ended abruptly when I crashed my mountain bike and sustained a traumatic brain injury.

Little did I know that my life, and the lives of those who love me, would be drastically changed forever.

The type of brain injury that I sustained is called Diffuse Axonal Injury. I spent the next seven days in a medically induced coma. My injuries included a fractured skull, a wedge fracture to my T7 vertebrae, and a fracture to my neck.

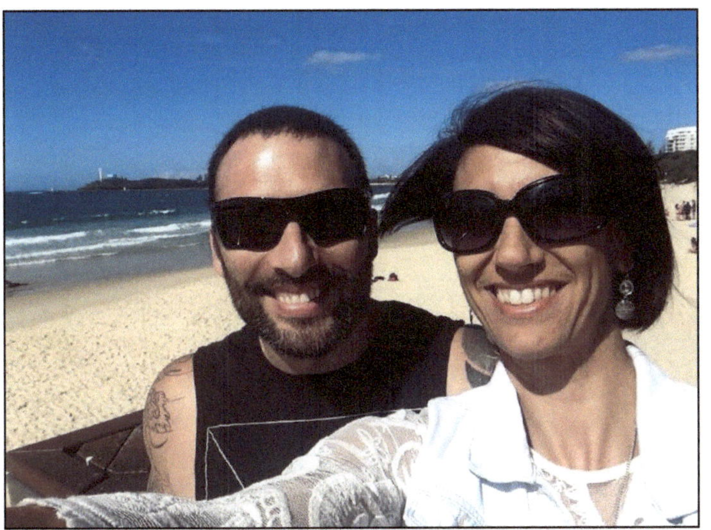

Post Traumatic Amnesia affected my memory to the point of having no memory of that fateful day, with the memory of my mountain biking accident forever erased from my brain. I cannot tell you where it happened, how it happened, the pain I was in, the ambulance ride to ICU or being admitted to three different hospitals over the two months that followed.

About the only memory I have been able to retain was of being discharged from the hospital. I had met the recovery expectations of the medical staff, so I was allowed to leave to continue my rehab and recovery on an outpatient basis.

I was advised by my occupational therapist that to help assist with improving my memory, speech and fine motor skills, I should start to write a daily journal of what happened, and what I had done or was supposed to have done during the day. To this day, I can't remember when I started writing my journal however, very slowly the words started coming out. I did the best I could to put them down on paper.

My handwriting was adversely affected by my brain injury. Before my injury, I had very neat handwriting and could write very quickly and legibly.

After my injury, my writing was the complete opposite. It was messy with numerous spelling mistakes. Just like my new speech challenges, it was not flowing easily or naturally. Using a computer brought no relief as I had forgotten how to use it and was suddenly unfamiliar with the keyboard.

I persisted with my new chicken-scratch handwriting, trying my best to remember and write down my thoughts. I don't know how long I had been writing my journal, though I think it was approximately twelve months before I could sense some improvement with my writing, language, speech, and concentration. My memory and neuro-fatigue were still the biggest challenges I faced. It was at that point that I read several books about TBI survival and recovery.

Prior to my injury, I had never heard or read about TBI. I said to myself, "Darron you need to write a book about your own TBI story as it will help you, but more importantly, it could help other TBI survivors and their families that are going through what you have gone through."

This is when my book, The Day I Broke My Brain, started on paper.

I re-read my journal notes as often as I could because I couldn't always remember what I had written. Diligently, I would pen chapter suggestions and topics to write about. It took me almost a year of writing. Writing a book was entirely new to me as I had never set out to do anything like it before. Like so much of life after brain injury, it was unchartered territory for me.

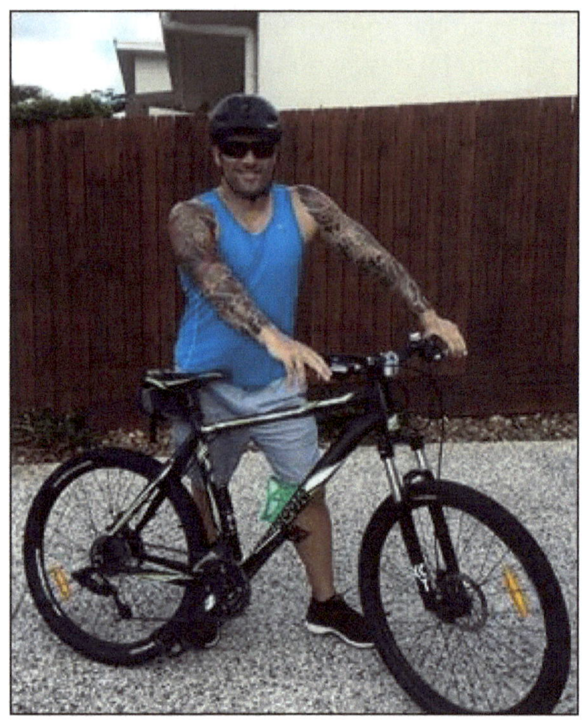

At this point in time, my story was entirely handwritten. I knew that to get the book project started, I needed to be able to email what I had written. My next step was to type up my scribbled handwritten notes so that I would have a readable format. I set myself up to type a few pages on a daily basis. I set myself a goal to have it completed within a month's time.

The typing was very much a form of rehab and mental stimulation at the same time. Though the overall process was very rewarding, after a couple of long days of typing I suffered from bad neuro-fatigue. It knocked me out for days, I was so mentally exhausted. This happened several times as I worked my way through the typing out of my book. I took the required breaks to help myself recover, and then I would start again. I was determined to finish.

A full month later, I completed typing the first draft of my upcoming book. The Day I Broke My Brain was born!

I was feeling really proud of myself, given what I had already been through. While writing my book, I was still recovering from my brain injury and all the TBI difficulties it brings to me on a daily basis. Writing my book is one of the most satisfying things that I ever have done in my life.

I still can't believe it really. I am actually going to have a book about my own TBI story. This is so exciting. The main purpose of writing my TBI story is to provide help to other TBI survivors and their families. My hope is that my new book may provide them with hope, motivation, and inspiration to keep positive and push themselves during their own recovery process. Readers may try something I did during my own recovery that assisted me, as it could help with their own recovery.

I have a framed quote in my lounge room. It was something I looked at regularly and read on a weekly basis.

It reads as follows…

"Sometimes the best thing you can do is not think, not wonder, not imagine, just breathe and have faith that everything will work out for the best."

I have used this statement as a kind of mantra to help me to live in the moment and not look too far ahead during my recovery. I still do it to this day. I believe that everything in life happens for a reason. I often say to myself that I survived my TBI so that my experience can help others.

At the time of this writing, I am almost two years out from my accident, an accident that gave me life membership as a brain injury survivor. My recovery is still improving and today I love my life. I hope to never forget that I am one of the lucky ones.

Meet Darron Eastwell

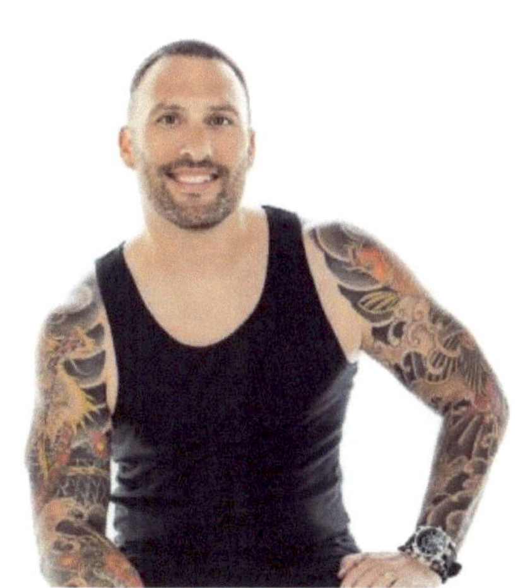

Darron Eastwell is a brain injury survivor from Queensland, Australia. The survivor of a 2015 mountain biking accident, Darron has emerged with a strong desire to serve those within the brain injury community.

His first title, "The Day I Broke My Brain," was released on Amazon in June of 2017. Darron and his wife Bianca share their love for their two children and have embraced their new life together.

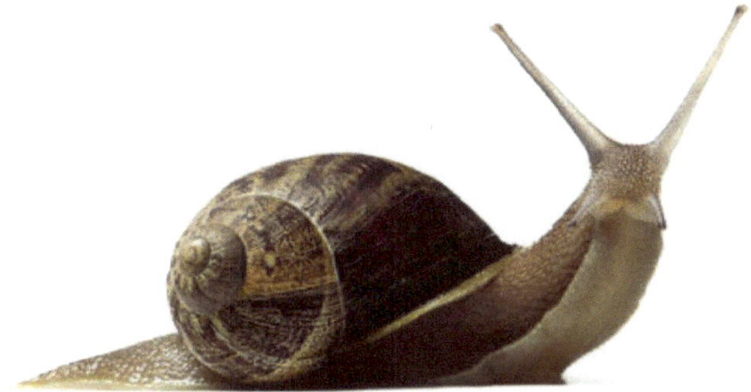

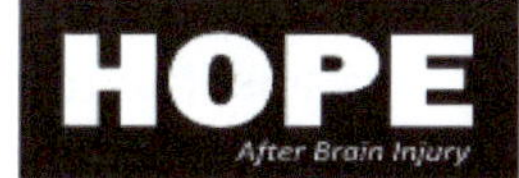

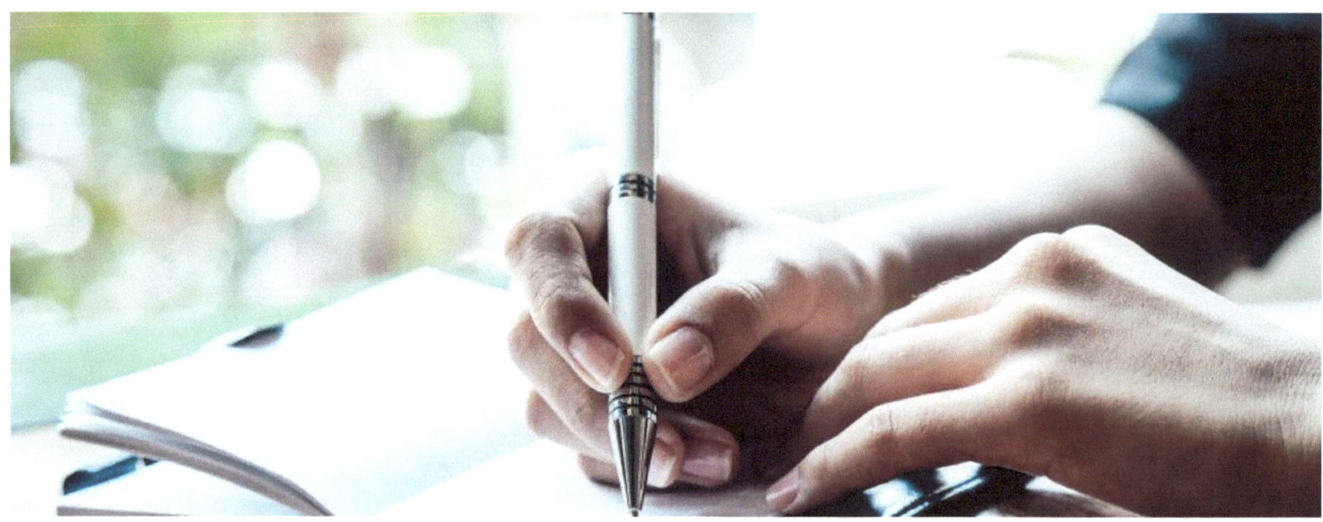

Journaling a New Story After Brain Injury

By Barbara Stahura

When a brain injury happens, the familiar story of a life can be altered in ways not possible with any other kind of injury or illness. So much you knew about yourself—the wealth of information you depended upon to lead your life—can blur or disappear, leaving you stranded and struggling in an unknown place. Along with cognitive and emotional challenges, you may face challenges with your physical abilities. You can feel as though you've been kidnapped to an alien planet where nothing is familiar, and you are lost in dangerous territory.

> "You can feel as though you've been kidnapped to an alien planet where nothing is familiar."

Family caregivers can feel equally bewildered, as well as terrified. I certainly did when my husband sustained a serious traumatic brain injury more than a decade ago. But my journal offered a safe sanctuary where I could pour out my deepest thoughts and feelings without judgment or criticism. Writing somehow made them more manageable. Despite being diagnosed with secondary traumatic stress, journaling allowed me to hold on and cope with the overpowering uncertainty, fear, and anxiety.

As I've found during eight years of guiding journaling groups for people with brain injury and family caregivers, telling your story through journaling can enhance the healing process. "Healing" here does not mean restoring your injured brain to its former functioning or your life to the way it used to be. Instead, it means finding healthy ways to become aware of, accept, and acknowledge what has happened so that you can move forward into your new post-injury story. Journaling, for even five or ten minutes at a time on a regular basis, can help release you from yearning for the past and open positive doors to your envisioned future.

How to Journal

There are no rules in journaling, except perhaps to date all your entries. So don't worry about correct spelling, grammar, or punctuation. You need not be a "good" writer. Simply write in whatever way is comfortable for you. You can write on paper or use a keyboard. If a brain injury prohibits you from doing either, you can speak your entries into a recording device, use speech-recognition software, or find a trusted confidante who will scribe your words without judgment or changes.

Keeping your journal private allows you to write honestly. But if you occasionally write an entry that you never want anyone to read, you can tear it out and destroy it. The benefit of journaling comes in the writing, not in preserving what you write.

To begin, you can simply pick up your pen or put your hands on the keyboard. But it's helpful to create a structure for yourself by starting with a prompt (for example: Today I feel… or, The most important thing I can do now…) You can experiment with various techniques such as Dialogue or Unsent Letter, or even setting a time limit.

If you're writing about a traumatic experience, don't simply begin writing with no structure in place. Even something as simple as a five-minute limit can help you avoid writing yourself off an emotional cliff with no way back to safety. Stop writing if you feel yourself getting unusually upset. And over time, try to keep a balance between positive and negative so that you don't end up endlessly ruminating on the darker aspects of your life.

After a brain injury, you might not be able to write much or for very long. Do whatever you can, and please don't judge yourself harshly. As your condition improves, you will be able to write more. If you're a caregiver, you might have difficulty finding time for self-care, but know that you can journal in only five or ten minutes at a time. A small journal will fit in a purse or pocket, and you can write wherever you are.

As you continue journaling, you will have written memories of your healing and of how far you have come since brain injury altered your life. And there, in those words on the page, you—whether survivor or caregiver—have created the foundation on which to build the new story that will carry you into the future.

Meet Barbara Stahura

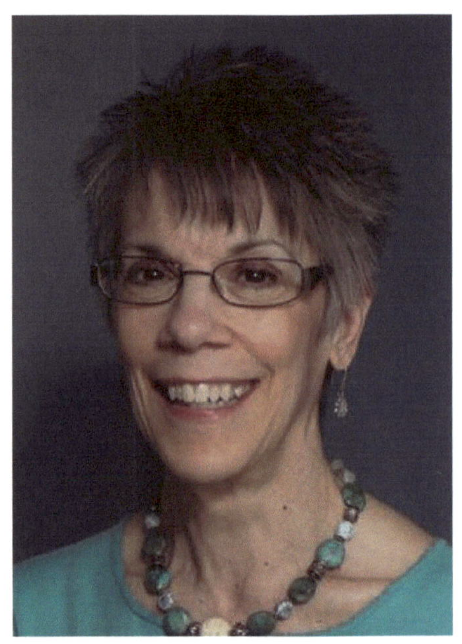

Barbara Stahura, Certified Journal Facilitator, has guided people in harnessing the power of therapeutic journaling for healing and well-being since 2007. She facilitates local journaling groups for people with brain injury and for family caregivers.

Co-author of the acclaimed "After Brain Injury: Telling Your Story," the first journaling book for people with brain injury, she lives in Indiana with her husband, a survivor of brain injury. To learn more, please visit www.barbarastahura.com

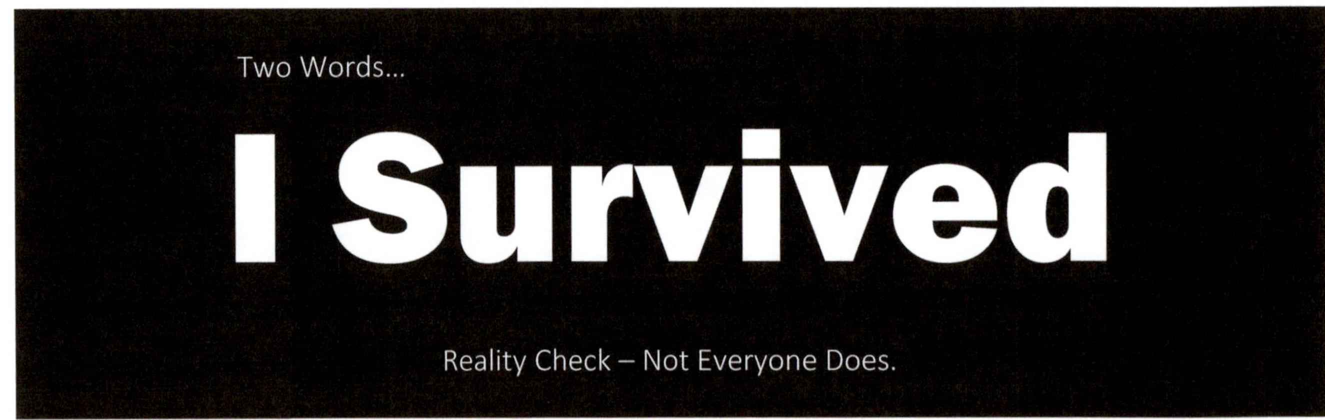

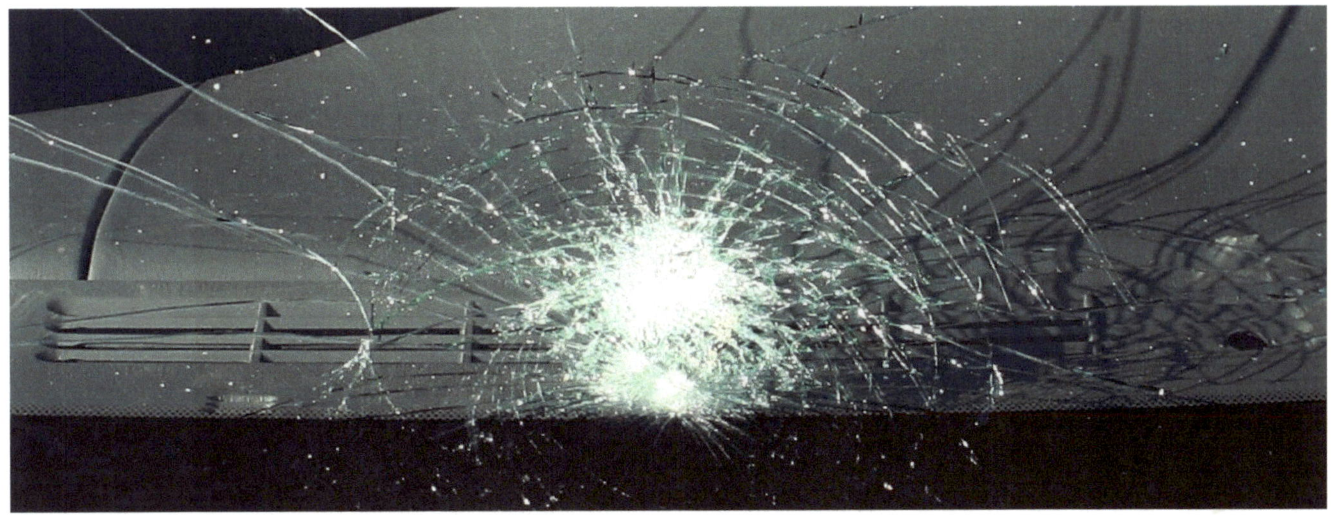

Suddenly Changed

By Dawne McKay

One week prior to my accident, I was on vacation in Florida with my boyfriend, and I was suddenly jolted awake in the middle of the night with a terrible feeling that something awful had happened to someone close to me. It was a feeling that I had never experienced before and I thought I was going to get a call that someone had passed unexpectedly. I carried this feeling with me for days and I just couldn't seem to shake this unsettling anxious feeling, no matter how hard I tried. Exactly one week later, I was involved in a horrific car accident.

I was on my way to work and had stopped to make a left-hand turn. I was rear-ended by an SUV clocked at 80 mph, and I was pushed into the path of a transport truck. My life as I knew it suddenly changed in a matter of seconds. I was transported to a local hospital, but my injuries were so severe that they had to transport me to a trauma hospital. When I arrived in the trauma unit, I remember being

greeted by the Chaplain as I was truly lucky to be alive. I suffered a moderate head injury with laceration, five broken ribs, fractured vertebrae, fractured finger and a horrific seatbelt wound on my thigh.

I only spent three days in the trauma unit, as they decided to discharge me even though I couldn't walk. I think back to that morning and I was actually excited to be leaving the hospital and couldn't wait to have a shower, wash my hair, and put my pajamas on. I didn't realize that I would be absolutely terrified to get into another vehicle, how bad the pain would be once the morphine had worn off, and suddenly

I realized that I could not walk, and I was in excruciating pain. Daily nursing, physiotherapists, occupational therapists, PSW's and numerous medical follow up appointments had now become my new way of life. Not to mention financial strain, flashbacks, sleepless nights, constant pain, the "what if's" and anxiety. I had a job that I loved and my social life and friendships as I once knew them came to a screeching halt. Friends who I thought would be there for me weren't, and I suddenly found myself realizing who my real friends were. (This is apparently quite common, as I talk to people in similar situations.)

> **"As I had never been in a motor vehicle accident quite like this, it was a HUGE learning curve and recovery for me."**

As I had never been in a motor vehicle accident quite like this, it was a HUGE learning curve and recovery for me. My accident happened in 2012 and I still continue to attend outpatient rehabilitation. I am still trying my best to cope with the chronic pain, sleepless nights and flashbacks.

Today and every day, I try my best to be as positive as I can, and I recently decided to create a Facebook support group for Motor Vehicle Accident Victims. I took it upon myself to not only build the support I was seeking, but to spread it out to others who were in similar situations.

The group has over 500 members, and a lot of them are either recovering from their accident or just starting to go through the process. Knowing you are not alone is the main thing and bringing people together and finding support in one another is very therapeutic. I find that once motor vehicle accident victims are discharged from the hospital, they really don't have anywhere to reach out to other victims. The group is strictly to provide members with emotional support while they recover physically, financially and legally. No medical advice, legal advice or solicitation is allowed in the group.

Meet Dawne McKay

Dawne started her career as a legal secretary and for the last 15 years has worked in the healthcare industry. In 2012, she was a survivor of a life changing automobile accident. She is the creator of an online Motor Vehicle Accident Support Group that went live in April of 2016. This is a closed group on Facebook designed to bring victims together to share their story, share information, resources and emotional support. Dawne's advocacy work continues.

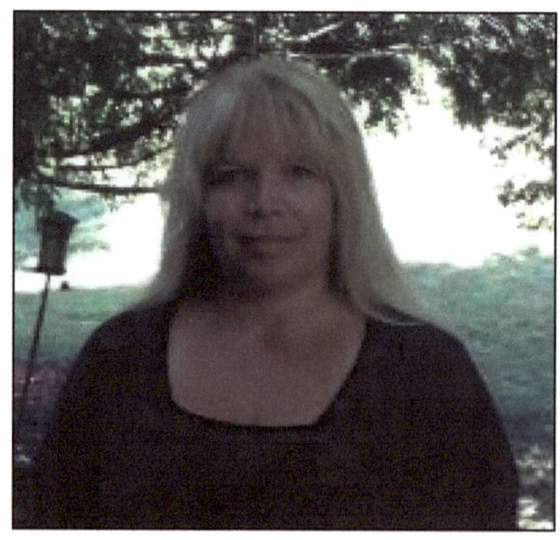

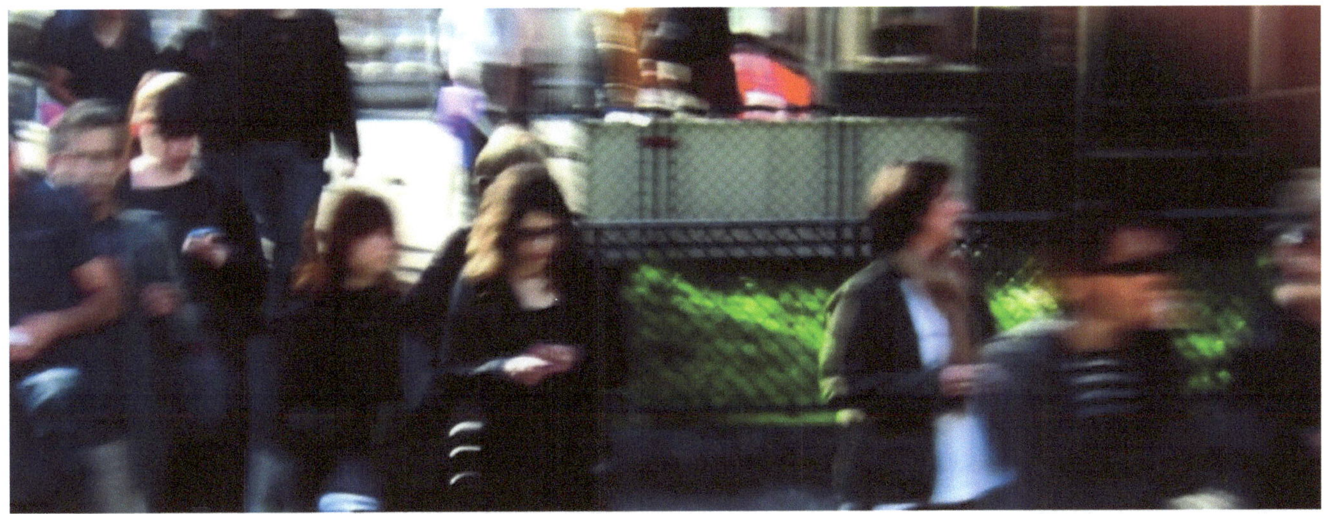

What Are They Thinking?

By Jeff Sebell

Sometimes people question what's wrong with us and say such blow-me-out-of-the-water unbelievable things that we are struck dumbfounded; unable to respond.

We are first made numb by the ignorance/unreality of what was just said. Add to that the fact that many of us have trouble processing information or shifting gears in conversations, and the result is we cannot think of, or articulate, a way to answer.

After a suitable amount of time has passed to figure out what actually happened, we might cry out passionately, "You don't understand!" and then get into some kind of argument. Sometimes, we might launch into an attempt to *explain*; always a bad idea given the heat of the moment and our exasperation.

> "Many of us have trouble processing information or shifting gears in conversations."

It Happens All Too Often

We take these things very seriously. When this happens, we feel as though our very essence is being attacked, and we feel a burning need to defend ourselves and clear our good name!

Only on those rare occasions when we are able to use all our power to restrain ourselves from impulsively answering, are we able to simply walk away, shaking our heads and muttering under our breath. We walk away, wondering how they could say something so ignorant, or stupid, or mean.

People's reactions to the things we say and the things we sometimes do; their quick quips and offhanded statements, reinforce all the bad stuff we think about ourselves. Rather than build us up when we really need a boost in confidence, other people often send us spiraling down into despair and depression.

It takes Two

Now, I am not making excuses for other peoples' behavior, and I am definitely not making it okay for others to do the things they do or say the hurtful things they say, but I do want to take a closer look at what might bring these things on, so that we may be able to see what we can do to help.

We need to take a closer look at the dynamics here. The situation is this: It might help us to understand why others behave the way they do, by first examining what kind of impact we have on **them**.

Interpersonal communication is never simple, although we tend to see it as simple. In our minds, we have been knocked for a loop by a brain injury and, while not necessarily looking for sympathy, what we are asking for is some understanding and support. Something to make our lives easier.

"What could be simpler than that?" we ask.

It Ain't So Simple

Let's look at the affect we have on others. Why don't we imagine you are walking down the sidewalk and a friend of yours comes up, approaching you from the other direction. What do you think is going through their mind when they see you?

> "It might help us to understand why others behave the way they do, by first examining what kind of impact we have on them."

Well, this person might be feeling uncomfortable, or have concerns or pity for this friend (you), who just doesn't seem right since his injury. Maybe he doesn't know how to be a friend in this situation and because of that, he feels like he is letting you down so he feels bad and doesn't know what to say.

In the end he just really wants to help but is not sure how. After all, he really doesn't understand why things can't be the way they used to, and this makes him feel helpless.

He isn't really sure what to do, and truthfully, some things this person says to you might be an attempt to "jumpstart" you, sort of like giving you a little, well-meaning "kick in the pants." Just something to get you moving in the right direction. He may not mean to be hurtful, but it comes out sounding that way.

Beyond not knowing what to do, there is a question of expectations. You are expecting support from this friend or family member who doesn't know what to do. You expect your friend to be there to help out as you transition to normal life, but even you don't know what that means. There are expectations and confusions on both sides, and a once-clear friendship with boundaries and structure is now murky and cloudy.

In my own situation, after my neuropsych exam, I sat down with my parents and went over the report with them in detail to help them understand what was going on with me. When we want others to understand but don't give them the tools, we are setting ourselves up for failure. The only thing that is really clear is that we cannot be relying on others to set things right in our lives. This is not their fault. The responsibility for a relationship cannot be all on one side's shoulders.

As frustrating as it might be, it is your responsibility to *teach*. Collectively, it is our responsibility to instruct.

Meet Jeff Sebell

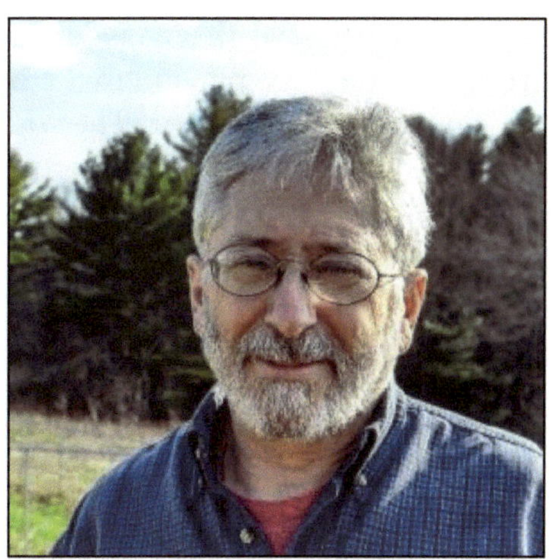

Jeff is a nationally published author, keynote speaker and blogger - writing about Traumatic Brain Injury and the impacts of his own TBI which he suffered in 1975 while attending Bowdoin College.

His book "Learning to Live with Yourself after Brain Injury," was released in August of 2014 by Lash Publishing. Jeff is a regular contributor to HOPE Magazine.

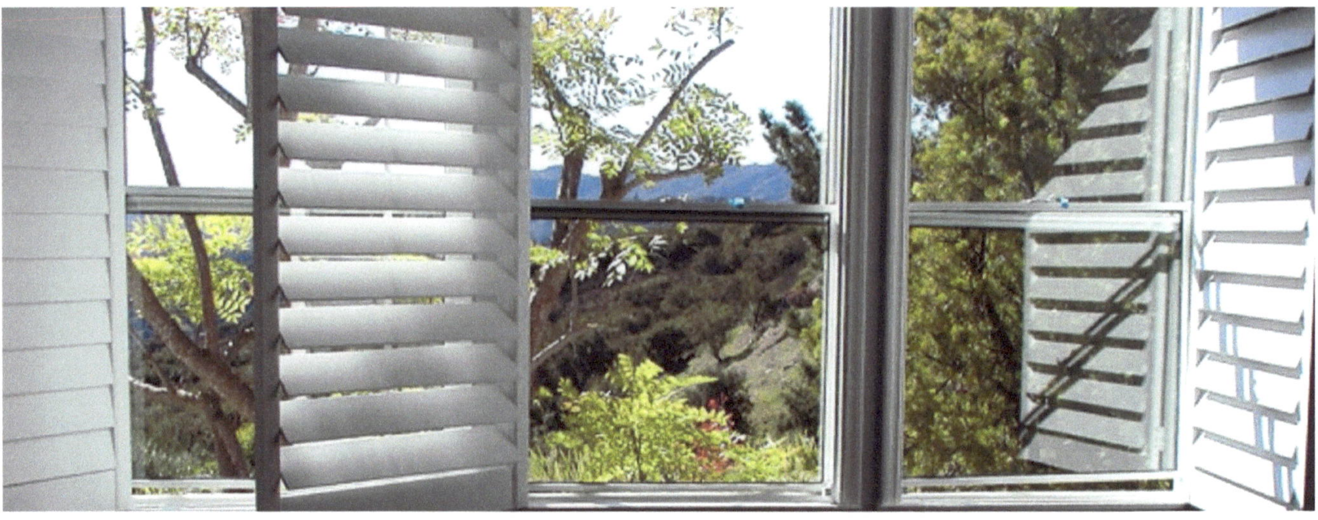

Colter's Story

By Mandi Seipel

Colter Pollock is an amazing, energetic, brave seven-year-old boy who suffered a Traumatic Brain Injury after a tragic fall from his second story bedroom window. On July 7, 2014, after a weekend of camping, the evening was supposed to be spent winding down but became our worst nightmare.

Five-year-old Colter was in a timeout in his bedroom after having poor behavior at the dinner table. At that time, his eight-year-old sister Jayden, and two-year-old brother Jaxon were playing in the backyard while I was cleaning up after supper. The sliding glass door was open, a slight breeze coming through and I could hear and see Jayden and Jaxon using their imaginations, playing away. Just as I was about to walk upstairs to talk to Colter about his manners at dinner time, the unimaginable happened.

> "I ran outside to see Colter lifeless and blue, lying on his back on the concrete patio."

I heard a loud crash that sounded like an egg cracking. Immediately, I ran outside to see Colter lifeless and blue, lying on his back on the concrete patio. Lying next to Colter was the window screen. Frantically, I urged my daughter to run and get help while I retrieved my phone and called 911. I was in such panic that I almost forgot my password to unlock my phone and even contemplated what number to dial. When the responder answered, I yelled my address and repeated it twice. At about this time, Jayden came running back saying our neighbors were not home.

While on the phone with 911, my hands were shaking so badly that I couldn't find the pulse on Colter's wrist. What I did know is that he was turning blue and was not moving. Just as I was hearing the sirens, Jayden returned with our neighbor Ryan Ostrander, who happens to be an EMT. He calmly and quickly performed CPR on Colter and affirmed that he did have a faint pulse. Some days, it feels like it just happened yesterday… raw but almost dream-like.

Later at the ER, we learned that Colter had traumatic damage to his skull. His brain was swelling, there was a bleed and he also had fixed dilated pupils. However, I had no idea what a brain injury entailed. We would find out that Colter suffered a Severe Traumatic Brain Injury, along with a

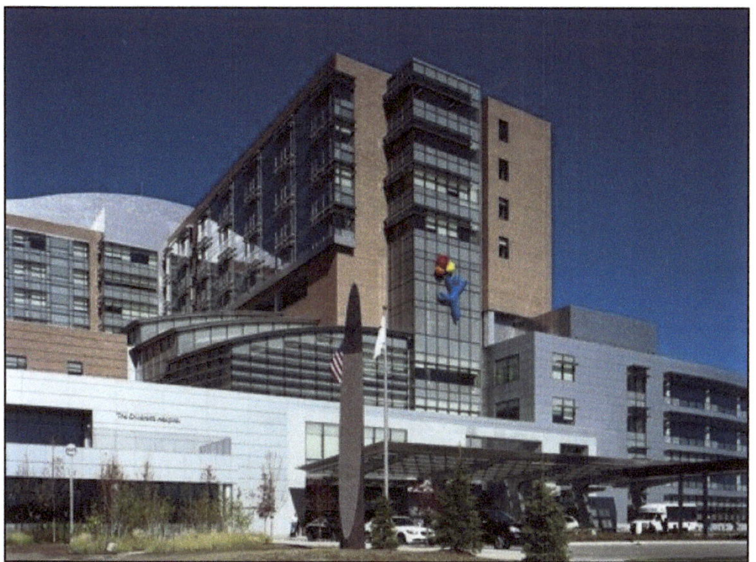

secondary diagnosis of left frontal temporal lobe contusion with a small subarachnoid hemorrhage.

After being life-flighted in a helicopter to Swedish Medical Center in Englewood, Colorado, I was told by his neurosurgeon Dr. Kimball, that Colter was a very sick boy and the chances of his survival were slim. He explained that Colter would need a left frontotemporoparietal hemicraniectomy for subdural hematoma evacuation to relieve the swelling in his brain.

The only glimpse of hope he gave me was when he said he had performed a craniotomy over 100 times and that he had not lost anyone yet. Signing consent papers stating that one of the outcomes could be death left me both hopeless and ill.

Over the next 4 months, Colter's journey became a list of unknowns. Miraculously, he did not break or damage anything else. However, the questions were never ending: Will he survive? When will he open his eyes? When will I hear his voice? Will he have his memory? Would he walk? How would he be cognitively?

Colter spent three weeks at Swedish Medical Center then was transferred to the rehab unit of Children's Hospital in Colorado.

It was at Children's Hospital where Colter began learning all of life's simple, basic skills. We basically witnessed all of his life milestones for the second time.

During many moments, it felt like he would never be "normal" again. But, what I did not know then is that not only is TBI an invisible, uneducated injury, but that he would never 100% recover.

Colter is purely God's miracle. While Colter was in an induced coma, Dr. Kimball said that Colter's life will be a marathon. In the past two and a half years I often come back to the word, "marathon."

Colter has defied the odds in his journey thus far. This marathon has not been an easy race. We have hit a lot of bumps along the way and are still learning how we can pace him on his journey. One of the hardest parts of his injury is that he looks and appears to be normal, and it is easy for his behaviors to be misinterpreted. Hard days are hard, but we are blessed and very proud of his achievements.

Today, Colter is a determined seven-year-old, first-grade boy who loves sports, is great at math and reading, and plans to grow up working with animals. Although Colter is defeating the odds, it's important to note that his journey of healing has not been an easy one. He has challenges and struggles that include his eyesight, sensitivity to light, perseveration, impulsiveness, safety awareness, headaches, and fatigue.

These are not closed chapters, but ones that are real to the effects of a Traumatic Brain Injury. We continue to not only advocate for window fall prevention but also raise awareness about brain injuries and preventable accidents. It is our hope that we can prevent these types of accidents from happening to other children and families.

Meet Mandi Seipel

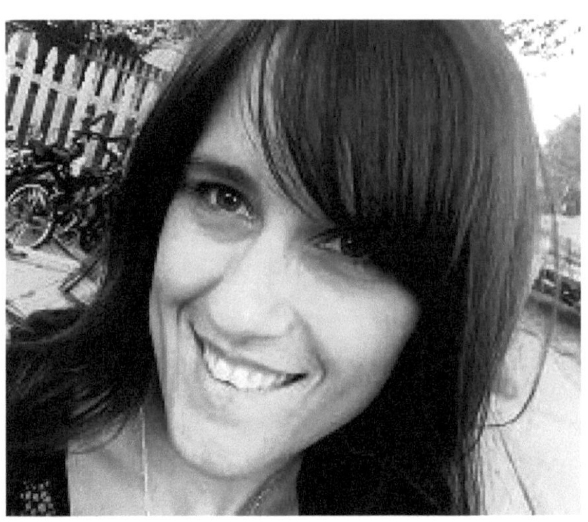

Mandi Seipel has been an educator for nine years, and most recently is a Title Reading Interventionist Teacher in which she helps kids improve reading skills.

Mandi continues her own journey with PTSD, while also learning more ways to help the whole family discover healthier nutrition and lifestyle choices. Mandi's determination will continue to raise awareness on both TBI and preventable accidents. She hopes to eventually be able to share her story and experiences to help others with their recovery.

"A hero is an ordinary individual who finds the strength to persevere and endure in spite of overwhelming obstacles." *~Christopher Reeve*

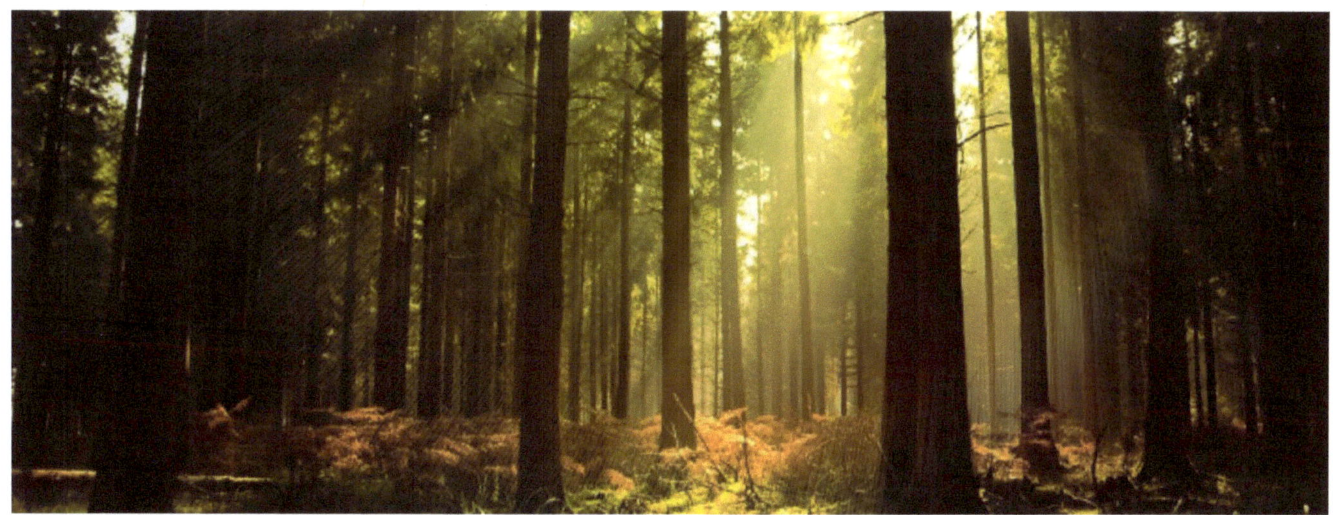

Two Life-Sustaining Questions

By Norma Myers

All parents are faced with the same common questions while raising their children. We were no different. *Will we be good parents? Will our boys be healthy? How will they do in school? What professions will they choose? Will they meet their soulmates and make us grandparents?* These are normal, casual, and expected questions until your worst nightmare becomes a reality. For us, the nightmare was a fatal car accident that took our firstborn son and left our only surviving son with a severe Traumatic Brain Injury (TBI) and a life without his brother, his best friend.

When we answered a knock on our door in the early hours of the morning expecting to see our sons, we were instead looking into the bleak faces of police officers as questions immediately started formulating. Because of the protective layer of shock that

> "In the blink of an eye for our sons, and with an unwelcome knock on our door for my husband and me, our family changed in a way that we could not even begin to comprehend."

consumed my body, I couldn't audibly ask the searing questions that I so desperately needed to be answered: *What caused the accident? Did my boys suffer? How long did they wait for help?* The agonizing questions kept swirling in my head, spinning like a washing machine stuck on the spin cycle.

The once casual questions of early parenthood turned into heart-wrenching screams, assaulting my heart like a machine gun stuck in an automatic mode. Unfortunately, some of my questions were answered without being voiced: *Aaron wouldn't get to experience the magical moment of saying, "I do!" He was robbed of the joys of fatherhood. No more hunting trips with his buddies. No more quality time with his brother. Family beach vacations for the four of us are now memories from the past.*

In the blink of an eye for our sons, and with an unwelcome knock on our door for my husband and me, our family changed in a way that we could not even begin to comprehend. While we didn't physically change addresses, it felt as if we had morphed into a new life full of unknowns. The chapter of our life as an intact family of four was removed from our parental handbook; in return, hospital staff offered a manual about TBI, and the funeral home handed us a brochure addressing grieving the loss of a child. These resources were meant to be a comfort, but all I wanted to do was find a shredder and do to those resources exactly what the accident did to me, tear them into a million pieces, with no chance of being put back together in the same way again.

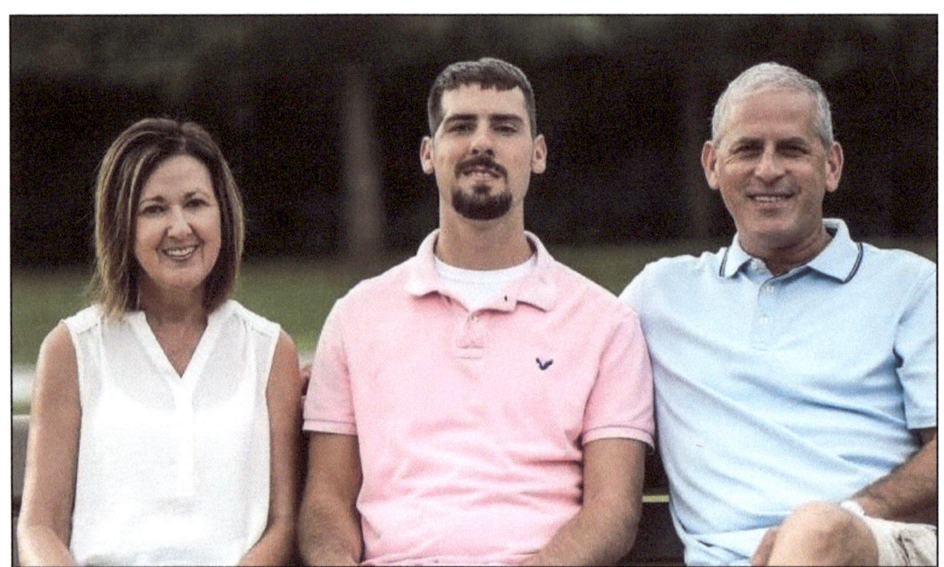

The merry-go-round of questions left me feeling queasy from the never-ending thoughts of what's next. The questions changed with each season of recovery coupled with each season of grief; *will Steven survive and what will recovery look like? How will I plan a life celebration for Aaron? How do I go about securing resources for Steven's rehabilitation and recovery? How does a family recover from such a catastrophic loss? When will we grieve? Will our marriage survive the greatest test of our thirty-two years together? Will our family, friends, and community continue to be there for us?*

As we watched our surviving son fight his way back to us, the recovery road wasn't easy. There were insurance battles. There were tears when therapists gave up too easily. And then there was our favorite: reminding healthcare providers that Steven could answer their questions himself, and on top of that, they didn't have to yell—his TBI didn't cause deafness. If I sound a bit sarcastic, it's because TBI has forced us to encounter the worst of the worst coupled with the best of the best. There are defeats that lead to tears and celebrations that are never taken for granted.

TBI alone causes a unique kind of grief, but when it collides with devastation from the death of your other child, it causes guilt for smiling. Laughter is followed by tears, not the kind of welcomed tears from a belly laugh, but tears from the remnants of a broken heart and ultimately experiencing a sense of sadness every single day, even when feeling happy. It's a complex journey.

I remember the early days following the accident. Amid the chaos, and despite the unknowns, my husband and I joined hands and hearts asking God to give us the physical and emotional strength to make whatever sacrifices necessary to ensure that we were by Steven's side providing security and support, all while doing everything humanly possible to keep Aaron's memory alive.

As we approach five years since the knock on our door, we are thankful that Steven doesn't let his TBI define him. We proudly watch as he sets, pursues, and achieves goals. TBI is an invisible disability; it can be very lonely if people are unwilling to get out of their comfort zone, become educated, and just show up. We are thankful for those that see beyond Steven's TBI and have the privilege of being exposed to his positive outlook on life. He possesses a *never-give-up* attitude and an infectious smile that reminds me of his brother.

Each day my heart experiences a tidal wave of emotions that threaten to sweep me off my feet. By the grace of God, I stay grounded, always asking myself two life-sustaining questions:

What would Aaron want me to do? What does Steven need?

I choose to believe that Steven needs and deserves the same mom he and his brother have always known, a mom who offers unconditional love, puts family first, forgives freely and never gives up. I know this is what Aaron would want.

Life goes on with traumatic brain injuries, with the loss of loved ones, with broken hearts, and unanswered questions. I am committed to remaining by Steven's side as he continues healing both physically and emotionally, and I will speak Aaron's name daily to keep his memory alive. I will continue to travel this path that was paved for me with grace and faith, trusting in strength that comes from God who so graciously restores my depleted strength daily.

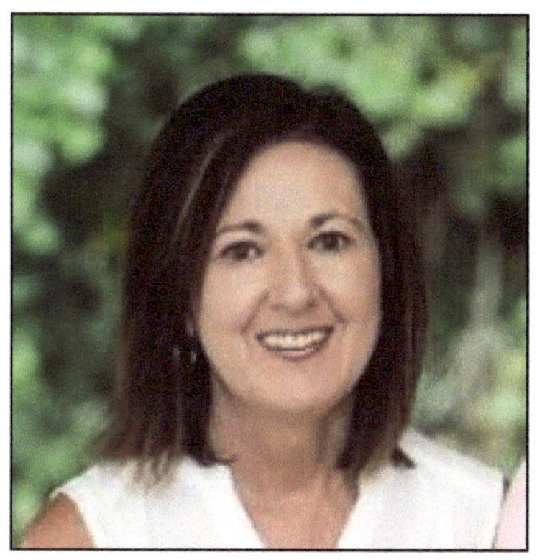

Meet Norma Myers

Norma and her husband Carlan spend much of their time supporting their son Steven as he continues on his road to recovery. Norma is an advocate for those recovering from traumatic brain injury.

Her written work has been featured on Brainline.org, a multi-media website that serves the brain injury community. Her family continues to heal.

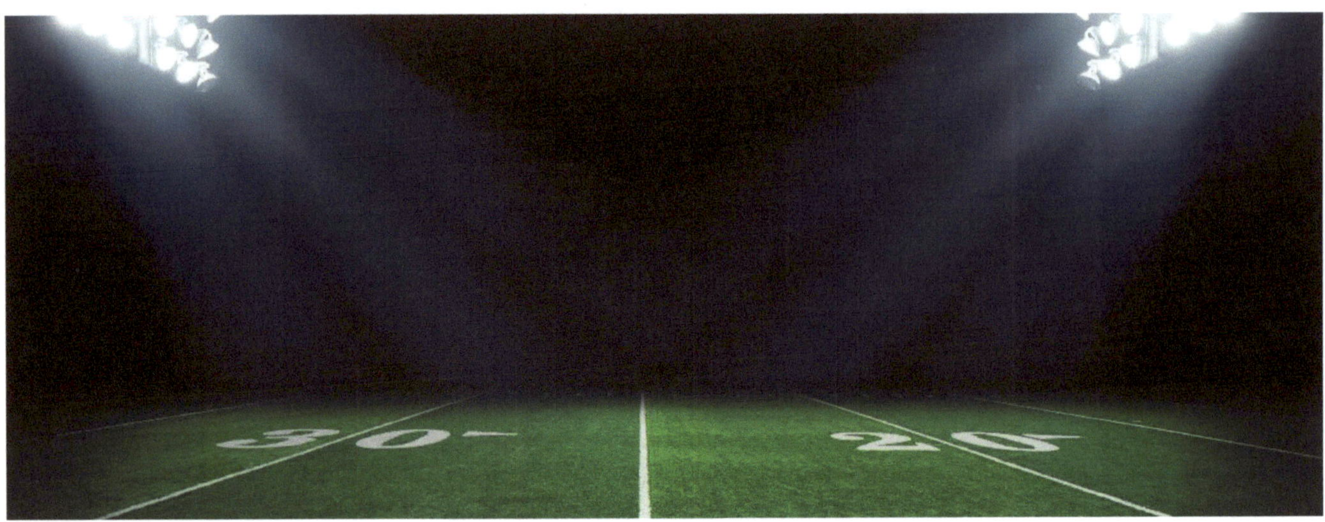

In the Dark About Sport's Concussions

By Ted Stachulski

Thirty years ago, my teammates and coaches were upset at me and confused as to why I just stopped playing high school tackle football. I had no idea how to tell them the truth and rumors ran rampant.

It wasn't because I couldn't get a ride to and from practices or games. It wasn't because I just woke up one morning with a plan to ruin all of my relationships and make myself an outcast. It wasn't that I wanted to devote all of my time to becoming an alcoholic and a drug addict. It wasn't because I wanted to end my athletic career on the lowest note possible after having devoted so much time and effort winning many ribbons, trophies, and championships.

> "I had racked up thirteen concussions from age four through age sixteen and got most of them while playing sports."

I had racked up thirteen concussions from age four through age sixteen and got most of them while playing sports. Football and soccer were the major contributors. When I was young, I went to the hospital after my first few concussions, but as I got older, I began hiding them so I could keep playing in games. I stopped playing soccer in middle school because of concussions. I should've stopped playing football for the same reason after winning the 1983 New Hampshire Pop Warner Championship Game, but I kept on playing in high school.

I didn't know how to tell anyone I had a concussion because I was brainwashed into believing that concussions didn't harm the brain and all I needed to do was suck them up like visible physical injuries. I was learning the hard way that wasn't true because after every new concussion, my symptoms were worse, and it took longer to recover. I was also learning that concussions had a negative impact on my athletic ability, academics, and relationships. I was losing the "real me" and I didn't like who I was becoming. Neither did anyone else.

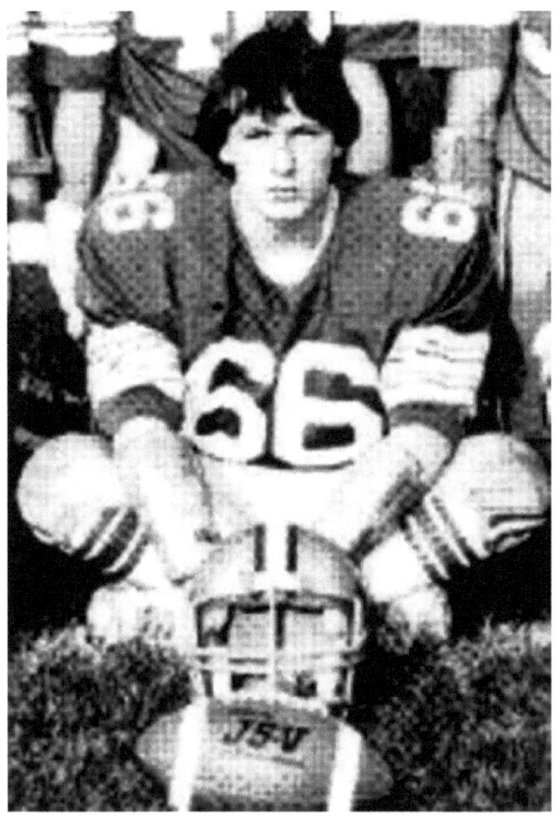

I was hurt mentally and physically from a concussion I got during a high school football practice. I should've told my coaches, trainer, teammates, and mother about the concussion, but I kept it to myself like I had done so many times before. To make matters worse, just days after receiving this concussion, I took to the field to play in the game. It turned out to be one of the worst decisions I've ever made in my lifetime because I injured my brain even more while making a tackle on the opening kickoff!

I was used to playing injured and thought I would always be tough enough to pay the price when the time came. No one should ever be so **in the dark** about **concussions** that they feel they can never give up or stop playing!

I lost a lot of friends and was ridiculed in the high school halls for abandoning the team. I had become accustomed to being called an Athlete, Offensive Guard, Defensive Tackle, Linebacker, First Baseman, Pitcher, Hurdler, Relay Racer, Sprinter, Defenseman, Forward, Captain, Co-Captain, All-Star, Varsity and Champion. For the first time ever, I was being called a quitter and even the people calling me that said it in a way that they couldn't believe the word was rolling off of their tongues. They were angry at me and I wasn't providing them with any explanation.

Suffering from Post-Concussion Syndrome and having no help with my academics, all of my grades dropped to F's and I dropped out of high school half way through my junior year. Also, I was engaging in risky behavior that was hurting me and a lot of other people. Family and friends tried to help me, but I was so depressed I just wanted to end my life. An uncle found me sitting on my bed all alone in the dark with a loaded shotgun held to my head. I am alive today because of him.

I was sent to the mental ward of the hospital where I had been treated many times for sports injuries such as stitches to the head, broken fingers, concussions, etc. This time, like the times before, they didn't want to talk about concussions and they drugged my mind into oblivion. I spent a month in a drug-induced fog. They released me back into the world in the worst physical and mental condition I had ever been in and just in time for football double sessions.

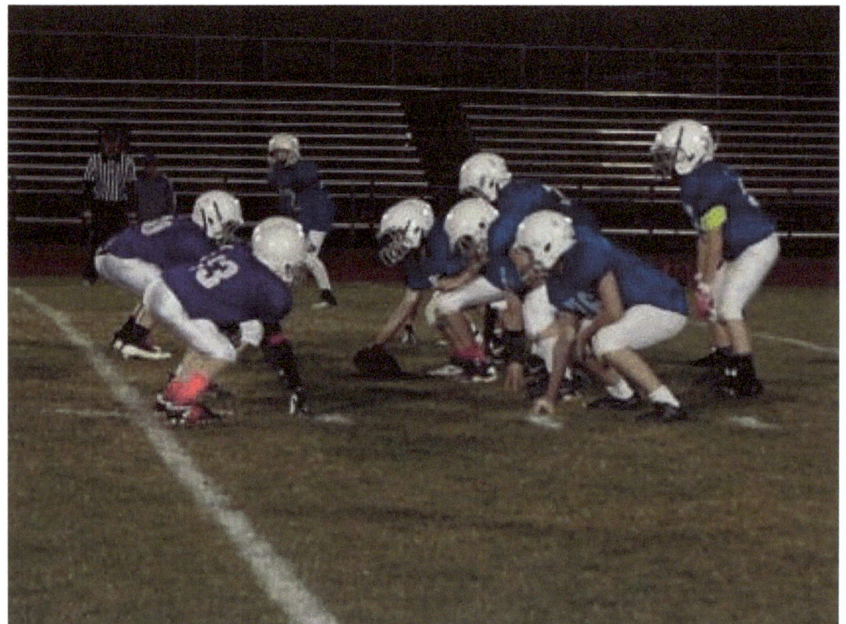

Even after all of that, I showed up for high school football practice for the 1986 season like an alcoholic looking for another drink or a drug addict looking for another fix. The new head coach looked at me and made me a running back. I injured my knee during a practice and didn't play in any games that year. Lucky for me, it gave me time for my brain to begin to heal and focus on retaking my junior year of high school.

Even though my sports concussion experience was 30 years ago, athletes are still following in my footsteps due to the same stigma and stubbornness I had in which I failed to realize that the brain isn't that tough, and it can't "suck up" the damage from repeated blows and concussions.

You Might Be Tough, But Your Brain Isn't!

People feel the risk of injury outweighs the gain of winning a starting position on a team, a game or even a championship. Well, that's not true when it comes to your brain and it's great to see many athletes are finally speaking out about their falls from grace because of concussions.

Athletes, parents, and coaches need to realize that brains are needed for other important things throughout a person's lifetime. That there are short term and long term consequences as a result of repeatedly bashing a brain into the jagged interior of a skull or forcing it to shear while the body dishes out and receives punishing blows over and over and over again during practices and games.

Along the way, many players lose themselves like I did. They can't stand the person they've become and some resort to committing suicide. It wasn't easy finding hope and I had to dig deeper than I ever had to before in my lifetime to find it. I just had to hold on for dear life not knowing what was to come next.

In order to have enough credits to graduate high school, I took on a full schedule of classes during the day and some at night. During that time I developed meaningful relationships with others that didn't solely revolve around sports. I became one of the first high school Peer Outreach Counselors in the State of New Hampshire and told my story to children in elementary schools. I went to the prom and had a great time.

In June of 1988, I received my high school diploma while I was attending Marine Corps boot camp. During my military career, I was meritoriously promoted and honorably served our country. I got married, raised a family and had meaningful employment as an Electronics Technician and a CDL Driver.

I created the Veterans Traumatic Brain Injury Survival Guide in 2006 to help educate Veterans, their family members, VA medical staff, veteran service organizations, nonprofit organizations and several federal and state agencies about concussions and traumatic brain injuries. In 2007, I received the State of Vermont Traumatic Brain Injury Survivor of the Year Award for outstanding commitment, perseverance, and advocacy.

> **"I continue to advocate for Veterans with Traumatic Brain Injuries, so they too can live long and meaningful lives."**

I'm 46 years old now and according to my neurologist at a Veterans Affairs Polytrauma / TBI Clinic, I suffer every day with "severe post-concussion syndrome (or worse)" from the cumulative effects of those 13 concussions and a few others I had received in my 20's and 30's. I've spent over a decade in rehabilitation for vision, hearing, balance, speech, swallowing, muscle spasms and other damage to my brain.

I continue to advocate for Veterans with Traumatic Brain Injuries, so they too can live long and meaningful lives. I've provided a lot of suicide prevention and saved a lot of Veterans lives by drawing upon my personal experience from 1985 through 1988. Those Veterans have gone on to help other Veterans break the STIGMA and get help for their INVISIBLE injuries.

Like Veterans, brain-injured athletes need a safe and supportive way of getting the help they need to heal and return to play or end their careers if they choose to do so. A healthy and honorable alternative to the old way of having stigma and peer pressure force them to play hurt, end their careers alone in shame or commit suicide.

I'm a member of the Krempels Center, a nonprofit organization located in Portsmouth, New Hampshire, dedicated to improving the lives of people living with brain injury from trauma, tumor or stroke. In partnership with universities and community volunteers, they offer programs that engage members in meaningful and productive experiences and provide ongoing support and resources to survivors and their families. The staff and other members participate in a group called "Man Cave," where we talk about men's issues and what it really means to be a man. I thank each and every one of them for giving me the inspiration to write this article which I've wanted and needed to write for such a long time.

After receiving a traumatic brain injury in 2001, I developed Post Trauma Vision Syndrome and Auditory Processing Disorder. My brain was over stimulated by visual and auditory inputs and it prevented me from doing many daily activities which people take for granted like going to the grocery store, sporting events and my children's concerts.

In 2014, my neurologist, Dr. James Whitlock, gave me a referral to a vision specialist, Dr. Kevin Chauvette at Merrimack Vision Care in New Hampshire. After forty sessions of vision therapy, I was once again able to see in 3D and listen to music as loudly as I wanted. It was amazing being able to make it past the second aisle of the grocery store and attend all of my children's school and sporting events!

I heard the song *"In the Dark,"* by Billy Squier on the radio and found it easy to put my concussion legacy to the words. I contacted Billy Squier and asked him for permission to use his song lyrics along with my commentary to raise awareness about sports concussions. I'm very grateful to him for giving me permission to do so. I hope our words together will educate people about the dangers of not disclosing and seeking help for sports concussions. I hope our words can help athletes out of a bad situation if they are currently in one like I was thirty years ago.

> **"I hope our words together will educate people about the dangers of not disclosing and seeking help for sports concussions."**

Meet Ted Stachulski

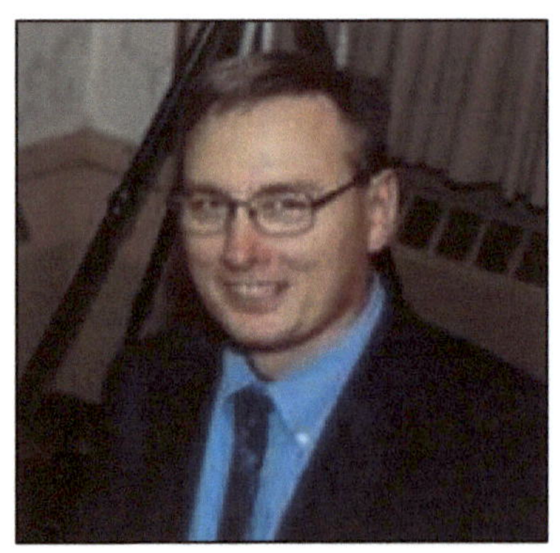

Ted Stachulski is a former multi-sport athlete, Marine Corps Veteran, Traumatic Brain Injury Survivor, and creator of the Veterans Traumatic Brain Injury Survivor Guide. Ted is also a Veterans Outreach Specialist and an advocate for brain injury survivors, their family members and caregivers.

From Us To You

Happy New Year!

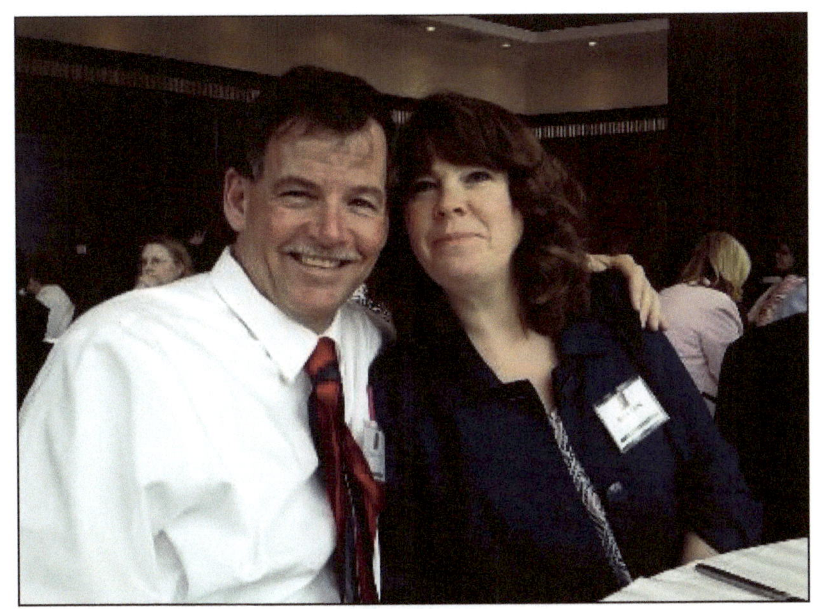

With Love,

David & Sarah

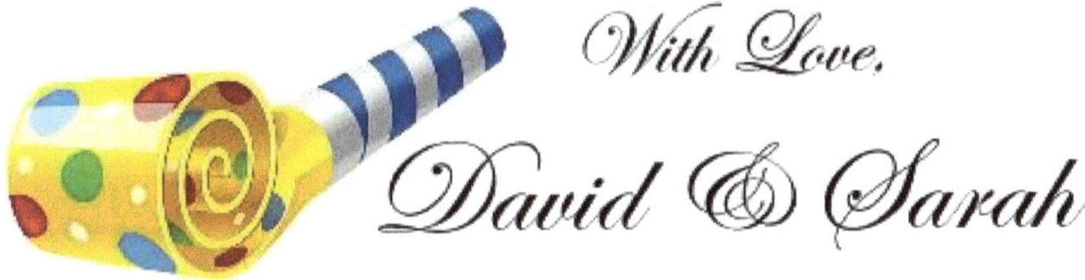